DIETS ARE HARD,

this is easy

A Practical Guide to Everyday Nutrition

DAVID RATH,

MA, RDN, LD

ISBN: 978-1984161437

CONTENTS

DISCLAIMER

This publication is for informational and educational purposes only. The information provided is not intended as a substitute for the care and medical advice of a doctor or other health professional. If you suspect that you have a health problem, you are urged to contact your physician/healthcare provider or local hospital for care.

SYNOPSIS

Diets are Hard, This is Easy: A Practical Guide to Everyday Nutrition provides all the information you will ever need to create a lifelong healthy eating plan for you and your family. Presented in an easy-to-understand manner by registered dietitian David Rath, this comprehensive guide touches upon every aspect of nutrition that you need to know. It assists you in making healthy food and beverage choices, but also allows for flexibility and personal preference. While written in a way that is interesting and personal, it also serves as a guide for various nutrition-related topics to be referred to as needed. Enjoy reading it as a book, but keep it handy to serve as your "in-house nutritionist"!

PREFACE

WHETHER YOU ARE TRYING TO LOSE WEIGHT, recover from a nutrition-related disorder, or pursue a lifestyle that ensures a healthy, high-quality life, this book will provide the means to accomplish your goals. It provides all the basic nutritional information you will need, and in a manner that is easily understandable and practical.

After providing nutrition information to patients, friends, and family for more than a quarter century, I realized that it might be helpful to consolidate it all into a book. Many of my patients, after having several counseling sessions with me, say they feel like they have just completed a course in nutrition. They feel armed with information that will aid them in making healthy choices for themselves and their families. Many had been through nutrition- or diet-related programs before and obtained temporary results. They, however, were not armed with lifelong tools that they could use to get, and stay, healthy. The purpose of this book is to provide the "nutrition course" to you that so many of my patients have received over numerous sessions with me.

I have found no more satisfaction than when my patients, after making significant changes in their eating and activity, tell me that they have never felt so good mentally, emotionally, and physically. They are amazed at how much energy they have. After years of not eating well and sedentary behavior, they had lapsed into a state of lethargy. They became used to this condition and, over time, resigned themselves to the fact that this was the way they were supposed to feel. Upon realizing that it wasn't, they were ecstatic! I wish I had a pill that would make someone feel that way for about ten minutes. Then I would tell them that, by eating nutritiously, you can feel this way all the time. This might be just the motivation needed to get them on board with a healthy eating plan. Well, since the pill has yet to be discovered, I figured the next best thing would be to write this book. I hope you will enjoy it and use it to meet your nutritional goals.

INTRODUCTION

FOOD IS CENTRAL TO SO MANY THINGS in our lives—weddings, anniversaries, romance, holidays, and other celebrations and social functions. Certain foods comfort us in times of physical or emotional dis-ease. This is why it can seem difficult when considering a change in how we eat.

I have fond memories of the "cracker soup" my mother made for me whenever I was sick as a child. While having minimal value in curing my ailments, the warm milk thick with broken-up crackers provided nurturing and comfort that made me feel better. I still experience warm feelings when thinking of her cracker soup. Remembering this provided my first glimpse at the strong associations we can develop with food.

We can, however, learn to enjoy healthful foods and beverages, while still allowing ourselves to indulge, on occasion, in the foods we have learned to love, even if they fall into the not-so-healthy category. What is most important is our overall eating plan.

When I was growing up, I never heard much about cholesterol, sodium, saturated fat, and added sugars. (Am I dating myself?) Breakfast consisted of my mother frying bacon and then cooking the eggs in the bacon grease. When eating corn on the cob, my family slathered butter on it and then salted it. We drank regular soda and ate full-fat ice cream. Then, when I decided to become a registered dietitian and began taking nutrition courses in school (in my mid-forties), I realized I needed to make some serious food- and beverage-related changes in my life. So, slowly but surely, I began modifying my diet. I remember the first time I ate corn on the cob without the butter and salt and realized how good and fresh the corn tasted!

Sometime after making these changes, I read a study in which people were given healthy diets for a period of time. By the end of the study, they were enjoying the foods they had previously said they didn't like. I was so glad to see this, because it shows that you don't have to be a nutritionist-in-training to adopt a healthy diet and learn to enjoy it. You can actually acquire a taste for healthy foods. And it can be done late in life.

Diets are Hard, This is Easy conveys nutrition information in a way that is understandable and easy to put into practice. Each chapter is independent of the others, so you can use this book as a reference and review the chapter that serves your purpose at the time. There is one possible exception—the first chapter provides tips on how to modify your eating habits. If you can understand how to do this, you should be more successful in applying the information in the remaining chapters.

Living a healthy lifestyle should not be considered a destination. It is not something temporary, but rather a journey that we embark upon for life. It greatly increases our odds of living longer and, even more importantly, the quality of life we experience in those years. Each of us should make lifestyle choices that are not only healthy but realistic. Doing so will ensure that these choices will last. Okay, let's begin our journey to healthy eating!

CHAPTER ONE:
Making Good Nutrition Easy

HABITS ARE THE FABRIC OF OUR LIVES. Think of the time and effort we save because of them. When we brush and floss our teeth before going to bed, we don't have to contemplate each action involved in the process. Once a habitual act is ingrained in us we no longer have to think about it—we just do it! And we do it efficiently and effectively because of the repetition. Establishing new habits takes a bit of time and effort at first, but in the long run it pays dividends far beyond our initial investment.

The following are "signposts" that may help guide you on the road to good nutrition:

- **Start small,** achieving small successes and then building on them. Pick the low-hanging fruit rather than actions that are more difficult. If I may borrow from baseball terminology, don't swing for a home run. Hitting a single is easier, so put together a bunch of singles to score.

- **Be specific.** Don't say, "I'm going to eat more nutritiously," as this gives you no guidance for what to do or how to measure whether you are accomplishing your goal. You might instead say, "I will eat at least three servings of vegetables a day," because this is a specific action you can easily evaluate. Either you ate three servings of vegetables or you didn't!

- **Have a support system.** Having friends and family to cheer you on is reinforcing and increases your chances of success.

- **Find a partner.** Doing things alone can be difficult. Find a friend, family member, or work colleague who is willing to buddy with you. If you commit to walking, going to the gym, or making healthy meals with another person, it makes it more difficult to rationalize not doing it.

- **List reasons** why you want to establish a new habit and post it where you see it every day (particularly at point-of-decision places like the refrigerator door, pantry, or office).

- **Write down the habit(s)** you want to create and give a copy to a "witness." Announcing your plan to someone else can strengthen your commitment.

- **List action steps.** If creating the habit involves complex behavior, think about and then list the specific action(s) you need to take to accomplish it. Breaking something down into clear, simple action steps makes it seem more doable and increases your chance of success.

- **Minimize temptation,** particularly while you are attempting to create your new habit. Don't make it harder on yourself and over-use your willpower muscle. Do all you can to put yourself in an environment that is in line with what you are trying to accomplish. If you are trying to adopt a healthier eating plan that is lower in calories and fat, stay away from fast food establishments. If you do go out to eat, find a restaurant that has plenty of appetizing choices that are in sync with your goal. And keep those cookies on the grocery store shelf, not in your pantry!

- **Know your triggers.** Be aware of what situations and circumstances (e.g. places, foods, and emotions) can break down your resolve and lead you toward the actions you are trying to change. Triggers can be avoided or minimized by the control you exert over your environment. For example, if you have a weakness for chocolate cake, it might be prudent to not have it in the house. After your new eating habit has been engrained, you may then be able to enjoy foods like this in moderation. If stress is a trigger to overindulge in foods of lesser nutritional value, try alternative responses—relaxation exercises, meditation, exercise, gardening, talking with a friend, etc.

- **Don't be discouraged** if you revert to an old habit. See it as a minor setback, not a failure. Each time you employ the actions relating to your new habit, you build upon its foundation. Then, when you reemploy those actions after a setback, they continue to add to that foundation. You are not starting over again. Eventually, when that foundation is strong enough, the new habit will take over and success will be yours!

- **Be futuristic.** Train your mind to see yourself in the future as a healthy, energetic person who feels great, physically and emotionally. Doing so will help diminish the strength of immediate gratification from eating that donut instead of a piece of fruit or watching television instead of taking a walk with a friend. It will also help you to develop a self-image as someone who sees the importance of health and lives accordingly. Then the concept of a self-fulfilling prophecy will work for you—you will become what you see yourself to be!

Some of these tips may resonate with you more than others. That's fine. People are different and have different ways of doing things. This doesn't make one way better than another, though a certain person may prefer it. Many different roads can be traveled to reach the same destination. This applies to lifestyle changes as well.

CHAPTER TWO:

Making Healthful Choices

THE FIVE FOOD GROUPS WERE CREATED as a practical tool for consumers to use to create healthy, well-balanced eating plans that met the US Dietary Guideline recommendations. Eating a variety of foods from all five groups helps to ensure we get all the nutrients we need for good health. When planning meals, and on subsequent shopping trips, you'll want to make sure that you include plenty of foods from each group so that you and your family are eating nutritiously.

But being in one of the Five Food Groups doesn't necessarily make a food or beverage a healthy choice. Some are high in fat, saturated fat, sodium, sugar, and calories. Honey buns reside in the Grain Group, and the Protein Group includes hot dogs.

You must be an intelligent shopper to decipher the best choices. This doesn't mean that certain foods can never be eaten. You just may need to limit the quantities of these foods that you and your family consume.

A person's state of health and stage of life may also dictate the types and amounts of foods and beverages they consume. For example, people with high blood pressure will need to limit their consumption of high-sodium foods more strictly than others. Children and premenopausal women generally need more iron than men and postmenopausal women. So, let's look at each group and learn how to determine which foods and beverages may be the healthiest choices for us.

Grain Group

Foods in the Grain Group are made from wheat, oats, rice, barley, and other grains. Whole grains can provide many B vitamins, minerals, and fiber. However, when grains are processed, the bran and germ are removed, and many of these nutrients are lost. Although artificially enriched with a few vitamins after processing, they are mere nutritional shadows of their former selves.

When deciding on which grain food to purchase, look for "whole grain" or "whole wheat" on the package's ingredient list. Don't be fooled by breads that say "wheat bread" or "multigrain" or loaves that are dark or caramel in color, as they are not necessarily whole grain. Processed grains not only have fewer nutrients but are absorbed more quickly, shooting insulin levels higher and making blood sugar levels less stable. Also, look for grams of fiber on the Nutrition Facts label, as the Grain Group is one major source of the fiber we should consume. Bread should have at least two grams of fiber per slice. Many grain products, such as packaged breads, are high in sodium, so look for those having lower levels.

Dairy Group

Foods made from milk are considered dairy products. They are a good source of calcium for strong bones and teeth. Most people should strive to get at least three servings of dairy foods a day.

Since milk comes from an animal source, much of the fat it contains is saturated. This is the type of fat that may increase your risk of heart disease. Therefore, it is important to make low-fat (1 percent or less fat) and fat-free choices. Cheeses are often high in sodium, so check for varieties having lesser amounts. Dairy includes products such as milk, cheese, and yogurt. Dairy alternatives—such as calcium-fortified soy milk, soy cheese, and soy yogurt—can also be considered part of the Dairy Group. Check the label to see if the dairy / dairy alternative product has vitamin D added, as some do and some do not. Vitamin D aids in the absorption of calcium.

Foods such as cream cheese, sour cream, and butter, also made from milk, are not included in this group because they have no appreciable amount of calcium. If you do use cream cheese or sour cream, consider low-fat or fat-free varieties due to the high saturated fat content. (Plain low-fat yogurt can often be used as a substitute for these as a healthy alternative.) Butter and other spreads are discussed in the fats/oils section.

If you are a vegan, see chapter 15 for dairy alternatives that can provide for your calcium and vitamin D needs.

Protein Group

Meat, poultry, fish/seafood, dried beans and peas, eggs, nuts and seeds, and nut butters (e.g. peanut butter, almond butter) make up this group. Dried beans and peas can also be considered in the Vegetable Group. This is because, in addition to their high protein content, they are derived from plants and have nutrient characteristics similar to vegetables. So, if you are lacking in the Vegetable Group one day, you can count them as a vegetable. (You can't count the same serving as both, though—that's double-dipping!)

You should make low-fat choices from animal-derived products in this group, as animal fat is highly saturated and may increase your risk of heart disease. Red meat (beef, lamb, pork) should be limited. Try to avoid processed meats (bacon, sausage, lunchmeats) due to high levels of sodium and, often, nitrates for preservation.

As in the other food groups, you should eat a variety of different protein foods. At least two servings of the Protein Group each week should be from fish/seafood. Strict vegetarians and vegans can choose dried beans and peas, soy products, nuts, and seeds.

Fruit and Vegetable Groups

All fruits and vegetables and 100 percent juices are members of these two groups. Vegetables are nutrient dense, meaning they have plenty of vitamins, minerals, fiber, and other healthy substances. They are naturally low in fat, sodium, sugar, and calories. Fruits are very nutritious but are naturally high in sugar, making them a bit higher in calories than many vegetables.

Vegetables are natural diet foods. They are very filling because of the high water and fiber content, while contributing very few calories. This bodes well for shedding pounds while maintaining a healthy eating plan.

The importance of variety is exemplified best by fruits and vegetables. Food scientists are discovering thousands of nontraditional nutrients in plant foods termed phytochemicals ("phyto" being Greek for plant), which can lower your risk of chronic diseases and disorders. Many of these compounds are pigments that give fruits and vegetables their beautiful colors.

So, eating a "rainbow" of colors helps ensure that you'll get a good combination of all these disease-fighting substances.

All forms of produce count—fresh, frozen, canned, dried and 100 percent juice. Canned vegetables often have sodium added for preservation, so you may want to rinse them in a colander for a couple of minutes before preparing them. This can reduce sodium amounts by up to 40 percent or more. Fruits and vegetables can lose some vitamins from processing this way, but they are still nutritious.

Although fresh produce is packed with nutrition, it loses small amounts of nutrient each day from the time it is picked. The average fresh fruit or vegetable in the produce section was picked about five days before you see it. Frozen produce is generally flash-frozen just after harvest, deactivating the enzymes that nip away at nutrients. Therefore, frozen fruits and veggies can actually be more nutritious than fresh (but maybe not quite as tasty). Dried produce is higher in calories per volume because the water has been removed from it. This means it is also more concentrated with nutrients per volume, so you can put some raisins on your shopping list to spice up your morning oatmeal with extra taste and nutrition.

Pure fruit and vegetable juice is also a healthy choice. Before loading your shopping cart, however, realize that fruit juice is naturally high in sugar, boosting its calorie level. Having no fiber also means that it won't keep you full for very long. Moderation is key, even with 100 percent pure juice.

Storing fruits and vegetables at the correct temperature and humidity helps keep them from losing their flavor, texture, and nutritional value. Always wash produce just before you eat it, not before you store it, and use water that is safe for drinking. Storage conditions can vary according to the particular fruit or vegetable. See the chapter on farmers' markets for specific storing information.

Fats and Oils

Choose monounsaturated and polyunsaturated fats to lower your risk of disease. Cook with plant oils like canola, olive, peanut, safflower, and sunflower oils. Beware of plant oil exceptions such as coconut and palm kernel oils, which are highly saturated. When choosing salad dressings, look for low-fat versions with unsaturated oils, as studies have shown it may take less of these oils (as opposed to the saturated ones) to absorb the fat-soluble vitamins from the vegetables in your salad. Limit saturated fats by choosing soft tub spreads rather than butter or hard-stick margarines. A good choice of spread is one with added plant sterols and stanols, substances that can lower your cholesterol. Avoid trans fats, which are denoted on the label with the term "partially hydrogenated oil." Trans fats may increase your risk of heart disease even more than saturated fats. Manufacturers are phasing trans fats out of their foods, so these fats should not be much of an issue in the future.

Tracking Your Progress

One trick I use to ensure that I'm getting the nutrients I need from the Five Food Groups is to use a bit of mental computation. When planning a meal or snack, I think about what food groups are represented by each food and beverage I choose. This allows me to keep track of what food groups are included, as well as those that are not. By doing this I can keep track of my progress, and be sure to consume the recommended amounts of foods and beverages from each food group by the end of the day. This may seem laborious at first. However, like other changes we make in our lives, once we do it for a while, it becomes a habit that we hardly notice.

CHAPTER THREE:

Grocery Shopping 101

THE FIRST STEP IN EATING HEALTHY is to have nutritious foods and beverages on hand. So be a grocery guru! Follow these tips to become a master grocery shopper. You'll feed your family healthy, well-balanced meals, and at penny-pinching prices!

Grocery stores can be healthy-eating heavens or nutritional nightmares. It all depends on how you navigate them. They are retail businesses that profit from selling you their products, healthy or not. It is up to you to determine what to buy for the health of you and your family. Use this chapter to make wise purchases at the lowest prices.

Plan First

Planning is important for most everything you do, and grocery shopping is no exception. Good planning can save time, energy, and money. Of course, to plan well, you need to be armed with some information, such as an inventory of what you have on hand, how long various foodstuffs can be stored and under what conditions, which grocery stores carry the items you need, what's on sale, etc. In this chapter, I will offer some guidelines to assist you in this planning.

Create a Shopping List

You need to have a shopping list before you even think about going to the store. Your strategy should go something like this:

- Determine what meals, snacks, work and school lunches, etc., you plan to prepare during the week. (Inventory your pantry and refrigerator to see what items are getting close to expiration and include them in your planning.) Check your menu against the US Department of Agriculture's (USDA's) Five Food Groups—Fruit, Vegetable, Dairy, Protein, and Grain—to help ensure that you and your family will be getting a well-balanced diet.

- Make a list of the things (foods, drinks, ingredients, kitchen supplies, and equipment) you'll need.

- Inventory your kitchen and pantry for these items.

- Make a list of the items you need but don't have on hand. You may want to create a grocery list template that is divided into sections (e.g. produce, meats, dairy, grains, oils, seasonings, condiments, household goods, snacks, sauces, kitchen supplies/accessories, etc.). Search online to find different templates and choose the one that best suits your needs.

- Have a copy of the list on your computer for future list making. Keep a current list on your refrigerator, so you can keep it updated for your next trip to the grocery store.

- Look for coupons, sales, and/or stores that carry these items at the quality you desire with competitive prices. Keep coupons with your grocery list so you don't forget to use them.

- This isn't on the list, but don't go shopping hungry! When you're hungry, everything looks good. Don't sabotage your careful planning and list making by leaving yourself susceptible to impulse buying.

Grocery Store Schematics

Once at the store, you want to maneuver it efficiently. Knowing the layout of your grocery store will enable you to find the items you need without unnecessary detours (and greater risk of impulse buying). Although not all stores, most are generally laid out with the staples—produce, bakery, dairy, meats—around the outer edges of the store, with nonperishables on the inside aisles. Beware when navigating the inner sanctums of grocery stores, however, as this is where most of the processed foods, candy, sodas, etc. lie in wait for you. Know what you want, know where it is, get it, and get out quickly!

Shop Smart

Don't judge a product by its front-of-package labeling. It is often a misleading marketing tactic to make the product look more desirable. Front-of-package labeling that reads, "Healthy Choice" or something similar, may or may not be a healthy choice for you.

The Nutrition Facts label is mandated by the Food and Drug Administration (FDA) and must be standard for all similar products. You can use it to compare nutrition information between items to discern which is the healthiest for you and your family. For example, if you are concerned about losing weight, calories may be most important to you, whereas if you or a family member has high blood pressure, then you will want to buy the product that is lower in sodium.

To put the quantities shown for various nutrients into perspective, see the Daily Values on the right side of the Nutrition Facts label. This tells what percentage of the daily quantity for a 2,000-calorie diet each nutrient represents. If the Daily Value is 20 percent, then one serving of that item provides one-fifth of a day's recommended amount.

Another comparison to make is one that can save you money. Check the "unit pricing" on the shelf, as this will compare prices of similar items using a fixed quantity. One item's price may compute to 9 cents per ounce, where another is 10.5 cents per ounce. If all other criteria that you care about are equal, you will want to purchase the least expensive product.

With a little calculation, you can also make this comparison using the product price and the total quantity of product the package contains. Store brands are often virtual duplicates of more expensive brand-name products but at a fraction of the cost.

Observe each purchase as it is rung up on the cash register, and review your receipt. Surveys have indicated that about 9 percent of sales receipts have an error of some sort (e.g., ringing up the regular price of an item rather than the sale price).

Finally, good grocery shopping times are weekday mornings and early afternoons. Shoppers are few and there are plenty of specials. Late in the evening is another good time to shop, as people are usually at home, eating dinner. If you want to avoid store traffic, don't go on Saturdays or just before dinnertime during the week.

Be Adventurous on Occasion

This goes against the grocery planning I just talked about. But sometimes it's good to nose around a bit and discover new foods and beverages that may be on the market.

The food industry regularly introduces thousands of new products, either reformulations of existing products or totally new ones. Many of these items cater to consumer interest in health and weight loss. Browsing aisles can help find foods and beverages that both appeal to our tastes and help us stay within our healthy eating plan, allowing us greater dietary diversity.

Understand what you are looking for, and resist buying an item just because it happens to be new or its packaging looks inviting. Scrutinize these new items in the same manner as mentioned above, considering the criteria of health, quality, and cost.

CHAPTER FOUR:

Eat Healthy without Busting Your Budget

MOST OF US WANT TO HAVE a little extra cash left after we've paid for life's essentials. We want to sock some money away for our children's college fund, save a bit here and there for a vacation, or just have a little extra on hand for a rainy day. One thing we can do to have discretionary income for these things is to keep our food costs down. Food costs are a major expense and can be a drain on our budgets.

Soon after starting a family, I began my career as a nutritionist. I wanted my family to be healthy, and now I knew how to accomplish that via healthy eating. Common thinking, however, was that it cost more to purchase healthy foods. Not having a lot of discretionary money at that point in my life, I began researching cost-saving strategies that would allow my family to eat nutritiously with minimal expense. Although my financial situation is much improved from that time, I still follow these strategies. I figure why pay more for food if you don't have to. I hope the information in this chapter will help you lower your food bills as well.

A little thought and planning can go a long way toward controlling our food purchasing costs. Below are some food budget survival tips that can help:

- Buy fresh produce in season. Check out farmers' markets where the produce is fresher and often costs less.
- Off-season produce is less expensive if you purchase it canned (in water or its own juice) and frozen. This way, you won't waste money having to throw away spoiled food. Canned and frozen produce is nutritious as well.
- Purchase milk (fat-free or 1 percent) in large containers, which generally cost less than milk in smaller ones. Nonfat dry milk is the cheapest way to purchase milk.
- Look for sales and clip coupons. Keep coupon and sales info in your purse, wallet, grocery list or somewhere handy so that you don't forget them when you go shopping.
- Shop at large grocery stores that provide more choices and often sell items at lower prices.
- Buy store brands; they are usually cheaper than, and just as good as, brand name products.
- Take advantage of in-store promotions.
- Look for the "unit price" noted on the display shelf, usually just below the product. This tells you the cost per a specified amount for different brands and quantities of the same item, so you can more easily determine which is the least expensive.
- Foods such as legumes and whole grains are much less expensive protein sources than meat, plus they come with plenty of vitamins, minerals, antioxidants, and fiber for good health. Also, consider nut butters, such as peanut or almond butter.
- Extend meat by putting it in casseroles and stews. These types of dishes (as well as other foods high in fiber and water, such as

fruits and vegetables) can fill you up with nutritious food at little cost.

- Buy nonperishable foods in bulk, and freeze unused portions for future meals.
- Clearly label foods in the refrigerator and freezer, so that you use them before they spoil.
- Go the "whole" way. Buy a whole chicken, cut it up, and freeze what you don't use for future meals. This is generally less expensive than buying precut chicken parts.
- Serve appropriate portions to avoid waste.
- Promptly refrigerate leftovers and reuse within a few days.
- Plan ahead so that you buy only what you need for meals, to avoid waste and unnecessary purchases. Check for items you already have on hand, then make a shopping list and stick to it.
- Don't go shopping hungry, or everything will look good, and you'll buy more than you need.
- Buy at a supermarket, rather than a convenience store, whenever possible, in order to pay lower prices.
- Spend smart. For the cost of bags of chips and boxes of cookies and candy, you could buy lots of fruit and veggies!
- Bring your lunch to work, rather than eating out—it's healthier and it saves money!
- Be a homebody—cook at home more often and eat out less. Check the Internet for fast, easy, healthy recipes. Studies show that meals eaten away from home contain significantly more fat, calories, and sodium than those eaten at home. Eating at home also gives the family an opportunity to spend more time together.

With just a little planning and shopping smarts you can eat healthy without ravaging your bank account. And then you can use the savings to purchase that gym membership you've been thinking about!

CHAPTER FIVE:

Healthy Food Preparation

YOU WENT TO THE GROCERY STORE and brought home loads of fruits and vegetables, whole grains, and other healthy foods. Now comes the tricky part. You must prepare all these foods you've bought.

When preparing them for meals, keep them healthy by not adding lots of extra fat, calories, sodium, and sugar. Often recipes can be altered to eliminate some of these unwanted items. For example, when I make oatmeal I don't add the salt that is called for in the instructions. I find no difference in the taste, and the texture is just fine. There are many other preparation tips and recipe substitutions below that should aid you in keeping those foods you purchased healthy. Use this chapter as your kitchen helper to keep your meals nutritious *and delicious!*

Healthy Cooking Tips

- Instead of frying, cook low-fat by baking, boiling, broiling, or microwaving.
- Grilling is another low-fat means of cooking. Marinade meats first to keep them moist and tasty. This also keeps them from getting too hot, so they don't release substances that can cause cancer. When meat is burnt, a chemical reaction is caused that creates a potentially cancerous substance in the black, charred portion.
- Keep the skin on poultry to keep the meat moist, but be sure and remove it before you serve it. The fat under the skin won't be absorbed by the meat during cooking.
- Cool gravies and soups, and skim off the fat prior to reheating.

Other Ways to Cut Fat and/or Calories

- Instead of butter and sour cream, add salsa, pepper, and raw veggies to baked potatoes.
- Use low-fat or fat-free condiments (mustard, ketchup, pepper, light or fat-free mayonnaise) and salad dressings.
- Fruits and vegetables
    - Steam veggies. You can use a pot with a steamer insert on the stove or purchase an inexpensive, microwaveable plastic steamer online for seven to ten dollars. The microwave option is quick and easy for both preparation and cleanup. Microwave time for steaming vegetables is about four minutes.
    - Oven-bake French fries and breaded onion rings rather than frying them. Coat them lightly with vegetable oil spray, then roast them in the oven at 400 degrees for about fifteen minutes until they're tender-crisp.

- Purée or mash potatoes and other vegetables with skim or 1 percent milk or reduced-sodium chicken broth, and limit the amount of butter or margarine you add.
- Purchase canned fruit in its own juice, rather than syrup with added sugar.
- Use low-fat salad dressings or make your own with less oil and more vinegar and limit high-fat or high-calorie extras such as regular cheese, bacon, fatty meats, croutons, etc.

Healthy Food Preparation Substitutions

Recipe ingredients aren't written in stone. You can use alternative, healthier ingredients and still yield great-tasting results.

Original Ingredient	Healthy Alternative Ingredient
1 large whole egg	2 large egg whites, ¼ cup egg whites or commercial egg substitute (use this substitution for ½ the eggs if baking, or product may be less tender)
Whole milk	Skim or 1 percent milk (optional: may want to add 1 tablespoon of vegetable oil for better result, depending on what you are preparing)
1 cup heavy cream	1 cup evaporated skim milk, light cream or half & half
Sour cream	Low-fat or fat-free sour cream
Cottage cheese	Low-fat cottage cheese
Full-fat cheese	Reduced-fat cheese (don't use nonfat in cooking because it doesn't melt)

Original Ingredient	Healthy Alternative Ingredient
Butter, shortening, or oil	Fruit purée (e.g. apple sauce, prune purée) for half the regular product; for prevention of pan sticking, use cooking spray or nonstick pans
Soy sauce	Low-sodium soy sauce
Flour, all-purpose	Whole wheat flour for half of the all-purpose flour in baked goods
Mayonnaise	Fat-free or reduced fat mayonnaise
Sugar	Can reduce to ¾ amount (½ amount in baked goods); add sweetness with noncaloric sweeteners or vanilla extract, nutmeg or cinnamon
Salt	Omit or reduce by half (except in products with yeast), and/or substitute herbs, spices, salt-free seasonings
Full-fat cream cheese	Low-fat or fat-free cream cheese, Neufchâtel or low-fat cottage cheese puréed until smooth
White bread	100 percent whole wheat bread
Iceberg lettuce	Romaine and other leafy lettuces, arugula, endive, chicory, collard and mustard greens, kale, baby spinach

"Healthify" Traditional Foods

Many recipes have been passed down from generation to generation. Indulge in traditional holiday fare or favorite comfort foods without busting your calorie budget. Just don't tell Grandma!

Original Food	Modification
Biscuits	Use vegetable oil instead of lard or butter, and skim or 1 percent instead of whole milk
Macaroni and cheese	Use low-fat cheese and skim or 1 percent milk
Cakes, cookies, quick breads, pancakes, waffles	Use 2 egg whites or ¼ cup commercial egg substitute for each whole egg (only half of eggs should be substituted in baked goods, to avoid tough final product); applesauce or prune purée to replace half of the fat
Dressings or stuffing	Substitute broth for lard or butter; add herbs or spices to enhance flavor
Greens	Flavor with skinless turkey, fat-free bacon bits, onions or peppers, instead of fatty meats
Gravies or sauces	Cool in refrigerator, then skim fat off top; use skim milk and light, trans-fat-free margarine for cream/white sauces
Sweet potato pie	Omit the butter and mash sweet potato with orange juice concentrate, nutmeg, vanilla, cinnamon, and only one egg

Making just a few substitutions can go a long way toward transforming an unhealthy meal into a nutritious and delicious one!

CHAPTER SIX:

Farmers' Markets: As Fresh as It Gets!

NOTHING SAYS SUMMER LIKE RED, ripe tomatoes and strawberries, juicy peaches and corn on the cob still in its husk. Summer is the season for farmers' markets to provide us with a variety of fresh, colorful fruits and vegetables, herbs, and a friendly, unique shopping adventure.

When I shop the farmers' market in my town I feel like I have access to all the area farms in one location. It's almost like being able to pick each fruit and vegetable directly from the field. I especially love the vine-ripened tomatoes, as they are so much better than the ones from the grocery store. My favorite fruit to get is peaches, when in season. There is nothing like a ripe, sweet peach that you bite into and feel the juice running down your chin. I also like the fact that homemade breads, jams, and other such items are often available as well.

I hope that this chapter will help you make the most of your farmers' market experience.

Planning Your Farmers' Market Visit

Find the farmers' markets nearest to you and go with your family, or take a friend, and make it a fun outing. It can be educational for your kids, helping them develop a better understanding of where we get our food.

Find out what days and hours the markets are open. Go early to get the best choice of produce. Walk around the market and compare the quality and price of the produce offered by the various farmers. You may want to buy your peaches from one, corn on the cob from another, and various other produce from some of the other farmers.

The table below gives an idea of how many servings you can get from the fresh fruits and vegetables in the quantities normally purchased at farmers' markets.

Amount Purchased	Number of Cups	Number of Servings
Berries (1 pint)	2 cups	4 servings
Cantaloupe (1 melon)	5½ cups	11 servings
Grapes (16 each)	½ cup	1 serving
Beans, green (20 each)	1 cup	2 servings
Broccoli (1 bunch)	7 cups	14 servings
Cabbage (1 head)	12½ cups	25 servings
Greens (1 pound)	9 cups	18 servings
Okra (25 pods)	3 cups	6 servings
Peppers (2 medium)	1½ cups	3 servings
Squash (1 medium)	1½ cups	3 servings
Tomatoes (1 medium)	½ cup	1 serving

Storing Fruits and Vegetables

You probably won't eat all the produce you bought right away. Fruits and vegetables can lose flavor, texture, and nutritional benefit if they're not stored properly. You'll want to store them at the proper temperature and humidity and avoid odors and gases given off by other produce stored in the same place. The items marked with * below are best kept in a plastic bag with holes.

Coldest Part of the Refrigerator (Crisper):

Apples*, blackberries, blueberries, cantaloupe* (after it is cut), cherries*, grapes*, raspberries, strawberries, asparagus*, broccoli*, Brussels sprouts*, cabbage*, carrots*, cauliflower*, endive*, leeks*, leafy greens*, lettuce*, mushrooms, green onions*, parsnip*, peas*, radicchio*, radish*, salad mixes*, spinach*, sweet corn*.

Warmest Part of the Refrigerator (forty-five to fifty degrees Fahrenheit):

Honeydew melon* (after it is cut), beans, snap beans*, cucumber* (after it is cut), eggplant*, okra*, chili peppers*, summer squash*, sweet peppers*.

Dry, Cool Place (fifty-five to sixty degrees Fahrenheit):

Garlic, onions, potatoes, sweet potatoes, winter squash, watermelon (uncut), tomatoes (at room temperature).

Special Produce Groups

Apricots, peaches, pears, plums: keep these in paper bags at room temperature for a few days until ripe (soft). Store the ones that are already ripe in the crisper. They are best if used within two days of ripening.

Cut melons: store them in plastic bag in the refrigerator.

Cherries, berries: keep these in a shallow dish and cover them with paper towels, then plastic wrap. They spoil quickly, so use them within a few days.

Mushrooms: refrigerate them in a paper bag or an open container so they get air. Cover them with damp paper to keep them moist.

Sweet corn: Store it with the husk left on. If the husk is removed, store it in a plastic bag.

Garlic, dry onions, and potatoes: keep these in a cool, dry place, separate from other produce, due to the odor. Do not wash them before storing them.

Ethylene Gas

Some fruits give off ethylene gas when they ripen. To maintain produce quality, store produce that gives off large amounts of ethylene gas away from produce that is most sensitive to the gas. Keep lids on storage containers.

Fruits that produce large amounts of ethylene gas: apples, cantaloupe, honeydew melon, peaches, pears, plums, tomatoes (ripe).

Fruits and vegetables most sensitive to ethylene gas: asparagus, broccoli, Brussels sprouts, cabbage, carrots, cauliflower, celery, cucumber, eggplant, endive, green beans, leafy greens, leeks, lettuce, okra, onions, peas, peppers, potatoes', spinach, squash, sweet potatoes, watermelon.

Wash produce with clean water just before using it, not when storing it. This includes the skin, even if you peel the produce, as bacteria can transfer from the skin to the meat during peeling. When washing, use water that is safe for drinking.

As Fresh as You Can Get! If you want fresh fruits and veggies, go to your local farmers' market. It's the next best thing to picking them from the field!

CHAPTER SEVEN:

There's No Place Like Home ...
Especially When It Comes to Eating!

WE NEVER FOUND THE WEAPONS of mass destruction, but unfortunately, the weapons of mass expansion are ubiquitous. Fast-food eateries and restaurants are everywhere and, according to surveys, people are eating at them more than ever.

Changing lifestyles account for much of this increase, which can be attributed to:

- Both husband and wife working.
- Trying to fit as much into our days as possible (work, extracurricular activities).
- Multitasking becoming the norm. We try to do more by doing several things simultaneously.
- Convenience. It takes time and effort to prepare a meal and clean up afterward. We just don't have the time and energy for it by the time we get home from work, not to mention taking the kids to soccer, dance, etc.

- The skills and knowledge are gone. More recent generations of Americans have grown up eating out and consuming packaged foods more often. They have not learned how to cook.

There are several reasons why the increase in eating out should be cause for some concern:

- Studies show that when people eat out they consume more fat and calories, and that eating just one meal per week away from home equals two pounds of weight gain per year.
- It is more tempting to make unhealthy choices when they are right in front of you, readily available, and emanating all the sensory cues.
- Restaurants encourage appetizers, desserts, and caloric drinks to increase sales, making us prone to overindulge.
- How about the bread/chip basket that's put in front of you while you're waiting for your meal? May as well eat it, right? After all, it's free with the meal and you're hungry. Well, the average basket has been found to contain about 1,000 calories. So, if you split one with a friend and eat only half of it, you've still packed away 500 calories—a meal before your meal!

There are also several reasons why we should eat at home more often:

- Studies show that children do better in school, have fewer behavioral problems, and are less likely to become overweight if they eat at least three meals at home each week.
- Eating together allows families to catch up with what's going on in each other's lives. Problems children are having at school are likely to be revealed at dinner—difficulty with schoolwork, being bullied, or growing pains. Don't use these occasions as opportunities to chastise or confront a child about something, or else she/he may develop negative associations with mealtime.

- Eating together can fill emotional voids that would otherwise go unfulfilled.

Even if you don't have time to prepare a meal at home, that doesn't mean you can't eat at home. Purchase a healthy meal to go, and bring it home for the family. You can also prepare meals ahead of time, maybe during the weekend when you have more time. Meals are then ready to heat and eat during the week. And you'll still derive all the benefits of eating together!

CHAPTER EIGHT:

Eating Out Healthy

ALTHOUGH EATING AT HOME has its advantages, many Americans find it difficult to do on a regular basis, due to increasingly fast-paced lives. Meal preparation is a lost art. According to recent surveys, many Americans no longer know how to cook.

I have many patients that often eat out because of their occupations or family commitments. Some have jobs that keep them on the road; others must entertain clients by taking them to lunch or dinner. Parents often have no time to prepare meals between work and getting their children to extracurricular after-school activities. Our sessions include a lot of discussion about the tips and information contained in this chapter.

Research shows that we consume more fat, sodium, and calories when eating away from home. Maintaining good nutrition while eating out can be challenging. It can, however, be accomplished. Below are some tips to help salvage your diet while dining away from home.

Fast Foods Chains

Fast foods typically supply a generous helping of fat, calories, and sodium, with minimal nutrients. However, many fast food establishments now offer a few healthy alternatives such as salads, baked potatoes, roasted or grilled chicken sandwiches, apple slices, parfaits, and fat-free or low-fat milk.

Here are some tips for eating fast:

- Choose charbroiled, grilled, or roasted sandwiches instead of fried. Avoid choices denoted by the term "crispy," such as "Crispy Chicken Sandwich" (crispy = fried!).
- Get lettuce, tomato, mustard, ketchup, relish, and/or onion on your sandwich and hold the mayo to reduce calories.
- Have a hamburger instead of a cheeseburger.
- Order a regular hamburger instead of a jumbo one.
- Avoid adding cheese and fatty dressings to salads. Most establishments offer a low-fat or fat-free salad dressing.
- Dress up your baked potato with salsa, low-fat butter substitute, low-fat plain yogurt, or pepper, rather than full-fat margarine, sour cream, or cheese.
- Drink skim or low-fat milk, juice, or water as a beverage instead of whole milk, milk shakes, or sugary drinks.
- Have thin-crust pizza plain or with vegetables. If you want meat, try Canadian bacon or ham instead of pepperoni, sausage, or hamburger. But if you are watching the sodium in your diet, be aware that Canadian bacon and ham, although lower-fat choices, are still loaded with sodium.
- At lunch, think "protein power." Protein makes you feel full faster and won't give you that afternoon letdown that you get with a high-carbohydrate, high-fat meal.

Restaurants

Dining in a restaurant does not mean you must surrender yourself to rich, high-fat foods. With a little planning and foresight, you can eat out and eat healthy as well.

Plan ahead and choose your restaurant wisely. Check restaurant menus on the Internet to see which ones offer plenty of healthy choices. If I know ahead of time which restaurant I'm going to, I'll know what I'm going to order even before the waiter gives me a menu.

But beware—healthy is often in the eye of the beholder! Whereas some people may be satisfied with an item that is low in fat and calories, if that item happens to be high in sodium and you have high blood pressure, then it is not healthy for you. See if nutrition information is provided so you can make this determination.

At all cost avoid buffets! If you go to one, you'll want to get your money's worth, which means you will probably consume many more calories than you need.

When ordering, you should:

- Choose broiled, baked, steamed, or poached instead of fried, au gratin, or scalloped foods.
- Request that gravies, salad dressings, toppings, and sauces be omitted or served on the side, so you decide how much to use.
- Choose whole grain bread or buns, bread sticks, English muffins, or small bagels rather than biscuits, cornbread, or croissants.
- Ask for (or bring your own) diet dressing and low-fat butter substitute.
- Choose meals with fruit and vegetables as main foods.
- Skip the appetizer and bread/chip basket (the average one contains about 1,000 calories!).

- Request preparation modifications. As a customer, you have the right to question how items are prepared and even request modifications when feasible. Don't be shy—you are giving them your business!
- Restaurants generally serve about twice what a regular serving size should be.
  - Split an order with a friend.
  - Eat half your meal and have the remainder put in a to-go box or, if you feel you may be tempted to eat it all, have half put aside in a to-go container before it is served.
  - Order smaller items, such as an appetizer (if there is one that is "healthy") and/or side dishes of vegetables (not prepared in fat) rather than an entrée.

Eating out with friends and family can be a pleasure. And with just a little planning and forethought, it can be healthy, too!

CHAPTER NINE:

Brown Bagging It

MANY OF US DO NOT HAVE the opportunity to leave work and go home for lunch. The best way to ensure that your lunch will be healthy and safe—and a lot less expensive than eating out—is by preparing your own and bringing it to work. It's also portable; you can take your lunch to the break room, outside for a picnic, or to a nearby park where you can walk around and fit in some physical activity.

When I worked at the state health department, I often brought my lunch. There was a city park just down the street with picnic tables and benches, where I would take my lunch and eat it in the fresh air while enjoying nature. After lunch, I would walk around the park. Not only was I eating a nutritious lunch and getting some physical activity, but also reducing any stress accumulated from my job that morning. Upon returning to work, I was ready to tackle the remainder of the day!

The following tips are meant to assist you with your brown bagging efforts:

- Plan your lunches; keep foodstuffs on hand for quick and easy preparation.
- Make lunches the night before, when you have more time; refrigerate if necessary prior to taking it in the next day.
- Have containers for soups, sandwiches, salads, fruit, veggies, grains, and other foods; this will allow for more options so your lunches don't become boring.
- Spice it up with gourmet condiments.
- Make sure to keep certain foods cold; if there's no refrigerator at work, use an insulated lunch bag and cold pack.
- Microwaves give lots of choice flexibility if you have one at work; if not, explore the possibility of purchasing one, possibly by employees sharing the cost (the same applies for a small refrigerator). We did this in my section when I was at the health department.
- Bon appétit!

You can also pack healthy snacks to have on hand in case you have a long period between breakfast and lunch or from lunchtime to when you quit working. This will ensure that you stay away from tempting but unhealthy vending machine offerings. Keep nonperishables handy in an office drawer and perishables in the workplace refrigerator or your insulated container with the cold pack. (I keep protein bars, trail mix, etc. in a sealed container in one of my office drawers. This will prevent the visitation of little critters such as insects or larger ones such as mice.)

CHAPTER TEN:

Surviving the Holidays
and Keeping Those Resolutions!

Being Merry *and* Healthy over the Holidays

Ah, the holidays! It's when you decorate the house and have good eats; invite friends over to have good eats; go to holiday parties and have good eats; open presents, then have good eats. Oh, did I mention eating?

Yes, we do eat, drink, be merry and consume plenty of calories this time of year—Halloween candy, Thanksgiving meals and leftovers, all the Christmas cheer in the form of food and drink (did you taste Grandma's fruitcake?), and those long New Year's Eve parties that provide so much time around the snack table (not to mention the alcohol, which is loaded with calories!). So how can one avoid the weight gain that seems inevitable, leading us to those New Year's resolutions we make that are so hard to keep?

Here are some tips to avoid weight gain and salvage your healthy lifestyle efforts:

- Don't show up to a party on an empty stomach. Eat something healthy and filling (like fruits and vegetables) before you go to avoid indulging on high-calorie treats.
- Keep your distance from the snack table. Engage in conversation, where grazing is not convenient.
- Do a sampler. Use a little plate and serve yourself a small quantity of each treat you would like to taste. (Don't bother with ones that are available all year. Concentrate on Aunt Martha's chocolate peanut butter balls that she only makes for the holidays.) Slowly savoring the taste will give you the enjoyment you seek with a limited number of calories. You won't feel deprived, nor will you feel guilty for eating too much. After you get your plate, move away from the table to avoid temptation.
- Imbibe lightly! Not only does alcohol have lots of calories but it diminishes control and increases the likelihood of indulging in more food. If you do have an alcoholic drink, consume it slowly and then make your next drink a sparkling water.
- Focusing on other aspects of the holidays, such as socializing with friends and family and traveling around the area looking at Christmas decorations, provides distractions from eating and drinking.
- Better yet, *walk* around looking at holiday lights, and get some exercise!

So, eat, drink, and be merry over the holidays. Just moderate the eat and drink part—be as merry as you wish!

Being More Resolute about Our Resolutions

Much is made of New Year's resolutions. Most of what I read and hear about them is somewhat cynical about their lack of success. Allow me to put a more positive spin on this long-standing annual tradition.

Sure, statistics show that after six months just over half of the resolutions made are forgotten. But that means that almost half are still successfully carried out. This is a time of year when many people indicate at least an inkling of desire and motivation to eat better and be more active, which is the first step in the process of change. So, let's say the glass is almost half full!

What can we do to make the proverbial cup overfloweth? Here are some tips that may be helpful:

- **Make a plan.** We all make plans every day. When confronted with a problem, we normally determine the steps that we must take to find a solution. At work, for example, we devise step-by-step plans to complete projects. We think about potential obstacles and barriers that we may encounter and decide how we will deal with them. Making lifestyle changes is no different. Think about your daily routine and determine where physical activity can fit. Maybe not thirty-minute blocks, but three ten-minute segments, or two fifteen-minute ones. Buy containers and foods you can use to pack healthy lunches for work. Purchase a microwave steamer so you can make quick and easy steamed veggies for dinner. Just a bit of planning and effort will help ensure success.

- **Make it a priority.** Just like other important things in your life, lifestyle habits need to be given high-priority status. One of the most frequent explanations I get from my patients for not being physically active is that they are under time restraints. After going over their schedules, however, we usually find times when they could fit in some activity. One recommendation I give to many of my "soccer moms" is to walk around the field instead of waiting on the sideline for their children to finish practice. One mom I know goes to a nearby gym while her daughter is at swim practice. Take a step back and analyze your daily schedule and find available times. After all, if your health goes, everything else becomes moot!

- **Start small.** Don't be in a hurry; this is something you want to do for the rest of your life. Small, gradual changes can more easily be incorporated into your lifestyle, as they are not as daunting as major changes from your usual way of doing things. Therefore, they have a greater chance of lasting until they become a habit. Slow and gradual is particularly good for a new physical activity plan. You are much more likely to avoid the excessive soreness and injury that can be a real show stopper!

- **Make it an adventure.** Have fun with it. Do physical activities that you like and will continue. You don't have to go to a gym. Join a dance club, Master Gardeners, a walking club—you get the idea. Take the time, when grocery shopping, to look for healthy foods and beverages that appeal to you. Learn about all the different types of foods and beverages that exist—they're endless! Make it fun, not drudgery.

- **Buddy up!** Find friends or family members who will accompany you on your quest for health. The more the merrier; you can reinforce each other. It's more difficult not showing up for your daily walk if you know someone else is expecting you. If you do join a gym, get to know some of the other members. The energy and support of others is invaluable, not to mention the fulfillment you'll derive from the socializing.

- **Make it who you are.** Visualize yourself as a healthy person. Practice seeing yourself in this way, and your self-image will change. Then the self-fulfilling prophesy will work for you!

- **Get help from professionals.** Be sure to get annual health check-ups from your primary care physician. Get with a personal trainer before embarking on an ambitious workout routine. Consult with a registered dietitian to learn how to eat a well-balanced diet to reach and maintain a healthy weight and get all the nutrition you need.

Following these tips will greatly increase the probability of success in accomplishing your resolutions. And if you're not successful at first, try again. After all, resolutions can be made anytime, not just on January 1st. Let's get that glass full!

CHAPTER ELEVEN:

More Energy ... Naturally!

WAKE UP EARLY. Make breakfast for the kids and get them off to school. Work all day. Take the kids to soccer practice/dance/baseball games/ karate. Get some type of dinner together. Make sure the homework is done. Get the kids to bed. Iron clothes for work the next day. Etc., etc., etc.

It's no wonder energy has become such a valued commodity! It is why we see so many ads for energy drinks and why we now find caffeine in everything from chewing gum to potato chips.

More than half of Americans drink coffee on a daily basis to get a dose of quick energy to meet the demands of the day. Using artificial means by way of coffee, energy drinks, and other delivery products to summon that quick burst of energy can take its toll. It is temporary in duration and needs to be replenished with more caffeine. It also uses up nutrients the body needs for other purposes.

Hectic, on-the-go, multitasking lives require that we be even more vigilant about lifestyle habits that impact both our energy and our health. These include

- Sufficient shuteye. Most of us need seven to eight hours of sleep a night to adequately recharge our bodies. Studies show that not getting enough sleep is associated with weight gain, and so another benefit we can derive from sufficient sleep is weight management.

- Regular eating patterns. Our cars get their fuel to function from gas, whereas we humans need food. To maintain a steady supply of blood sugar to fuel our cells we need to eat regularly. Moderate-sized meals and healthy snacks will provide a consistent source of energy.

- Consume enough of the right foods and beverages in a balanced diet.

  - Nutrients such as B vitamins and magnesium are needed to generate energy from the foods and beverages we consume. B vitamins, with the exception of B_{12}, are fairly ubiquitous in a well-balanced diet. B_{12} must be acquired from animal-based foods and beverages (see the bullet point below on B_{12} and folate). The mineral magnesium can be derived from whole grains, nuts, beans, lentils, bananas, and green vegetables.

  - Iron is important for carrying oxygen to cells for energy. (See the chapter on vegetarianism for iron sources.)

  - B_{12} and folate are required to build the cells that manufacture energy. Vitamin B_{12} is naturally found in animal products such as fish, poultry, meat, eggs, or dairy, while folate sources include fruits, vegetables, whole grains, fortified grains, and beans.

  - Complex carbohydrates found in whole grains, fruits, and vegetables are a necessary, steady source of energy.

  - Protein helps slow absorption, so that the energy from food consumed will be released more slowly, keeping our blood sugar steady. Choose lean meats, low-fat or fat-free dairy and plant-derived protein sources to keep saturated fat in check.

- Fiber from whole grains, fruits, and vegetables slows digestion and absorption for gradual, long-lasting energy.
- Concentrated sweets (e.g., candy bars and regular soda) consumed by themselves will release quickly, causing an immediate energy spike, followed by a letdown.

- Drink enough fluids. Dehydration can drain energy; fluid is necessary for body processes such as energy production.
- Control stress. Stress depletes the body of nutrients and energy.
- Have regular checkups, including your thyroid. A malfunctioning thyroid can cause fatigue; so can low blood sugar.
- Low T? Older men are at higher risk of low testosterone, which can cause fatigue. Only about 2 percent of men between the ages of forty and sixty-nine have inadequate levels, however. Have it checked by your doctor and get a prescription if necessary. Do not succumb to advertising that makes you think you need it and then encourages you to purchase over-the-counter supplements.

Finally, watch out for various herbs and other substances added to energy drinks, powders, and pills. Many products contain ginseng to "boost energy." The Commission E (Germany's regulatory agency for herbs) recommends no more than one to two grams (1,000 to 2,000 milligrams) daily of the root for no more than three months, because long-term use could be harmful, due to its hormone-like effect. Ginseng in babies has been linked to poisoning that can be fatal, and the safety in use by older children is not known. Pregnant women should not take ginseng because of animal studies that showed birth defects may result. Little is known about its effects on breastfeeding, so it should be avoided. Check with your health professional before taking any herbal products, as many can interfere with certain medications and disease treatments.

Bottom line: There's nothing wrong with moderate caffeine intake from coffee, colas, chocolate, etc. But when it comes to fueling the body, the best bet, health-wise, is to do it "naturally"!

CHAPTER TWELVE:

Nutrition for Exercisers and Athletes

WHEN I WAS AT THE OLYMPIC TRAINING CENTER in Colorado Springs back in the early 1990s, they had no dietitian on staff, nor did they have a nutritional strategy for the training table that they offered to athletes at mealtimes. This has drastically changed over the past twenty-five years, due to research showing the benefits of nutrition for optimal performance. Professional sports teams, major college athletic programs, and Olympic teams now have dietitians on staff to advise athletes on how to eat, taking into account the sport they are participating in and their individual preferences.

Whether you are a competitive athlete or someone just wanting to get the most from your workout, proper nutrition can make a big difference. Knowing what to eat and when to eat it can propel you to the next level in your fitness and performance. Let's start at the beginning.

Pre-Competition Eating

Pre-competition eating can be crucial to performance. If the body does not have maximal storage of carbohydrate energy (stored as glycogen), premature fatigue will result. No more than six hours should elapse from the time of the last meal to the start of the competition.

Composition

A high-carbohydrate meal is best prior to activity. Besides being the quickest and most efficient source of energy, it provides water for hydration (carbohydrate is about 75 percent water). Fat and fiber should be restricted to ensure optimal digestion. Protein that is low in fat should be eaten in small amounts. Large amounts of protein can cause dehydration. Liquid meal replacements may be a good choice if solid food ingestion is problematic due to pre-competition anxiety or other malabsorption issues.

Timing

Large meals should have at least four hours to digest, while smaller ones require two to three hours. Liquid meals need only an hour or two, and small snacks possibly less than an hour. A good general guideline to follow is to consume one to 4.5 grams of carbohydrate per kilogram of body weight, one to four hours prior to competition (the closer to competition, the smaller the amount of carbohydrate ingested).

To determine your weight in kilograms (kg), divide your weight in pounds by 2.2 (there are 2.2 pounds in one kilogram). For example, if you weigh 165 pounds, divide 165 by 2.2 and you get your weight in kilograms (165/2.2 = 75 kilograms).

Do No Harm

Probably the most important statement that can be made about the pre-competition meal is "Try to do no harm." Athletes should evaluate their responses to high-carbohydrate foods with both low and high glycemic indexes. Although high-glycemic-index foods can cause low blood glucose due to insulin spike, it is usually transient and doesn't adversely affect performance. Some athletes are more sensitive, however, and may need to consume a lower-glycemic-index carbohydrate before activity or wait until just before activity to eat higher-glycemic-index carbohydrates (the onset of activity will blunt insulin release). Gas-forming foods such as dried beans, cabbage, onions, radishes, cauliflower, and turnips can cause discomfort, so avoid them.

Individual Tolerances

People react differently to dietary regimens. Some individuals can eat closer to competition than others. Foods that one person can tolerate may cause discomfort in another. It is not wise to test new foods prior to competition. Many athletes have favorite foods that they feel give them an edge. If an individual has a strong personal preference for a food, the food should be allowed, if tolerated physiologically.

Eating during and after Competition

During Competition

Consuming carbohydrates (especially of high glycemic index) during a competition lasting longer than sixty minutes can increase endurance and sustain high-intensity performance by maintaining blood glucose levels. This can be achieved by taking in twenty-five to thirty grams of carbohydrate every thirty minutes through convenient, low-fat, carbohydrate-rich sources (e.g., sports bars or gels, bananas, oranges). Drinking sports drinks containing 4 percent to 8 percent carbohydrate every fifteen minutes will provide the appropriate amount of carbohydrate and satisfy hydration needs.

After Competition

Refueling your body appropriately following activity will assure that you have maximum energy to perform again soon. You should consume carbohydrate-rich foods and beverages as soon as possible. Including a moderate amount (about twenty to twenty-five grams) of low-fat protein with the carbohydrate will optimize energy replenishment, as well as muscle tissue repair and growth.

High-carbohydrate foods include grains, fruits, vegetables, legumes, and low-fat dairy products. Homemade smoothies or specially formulated commercial beverages may be preferred if solid foods are not appealing so soon after activity. An intake of one half to one gram of carbohydrate per kilogram of body weight, along with twenty to twenty-five grams of protein, should be ingested immediately or at least within the first thirty to forty minutes, if possible. This same quantity should be consumed again within two hours. Following this eating pattern can fully replenish energy stores within twenty hours. Also, be sure to completely rehydrate by drinking plenty of fluids.

Fluids and Hydration

Guidelines for Maintaining Hydration

The following guidelines will help maintain adequate hydration during training or competition:

- Drink sixteen to twenty ounces of fluid two hours prior to activity.
- Drink eight to sixteen ounces of fluid approximately fifteen minutes prior to activity.

- Drink at least four to eight ounces of fluid every fifteen to twenty minutes during strenuous activity (this can vary, according to climate, individual sweat rate, and activity type/intensity).

- Weigh in before and after activity. Drink twenty to twenty-four ounces of fluid for every pound you lose. (Thirst is not an indicator of replenishment needs.) Urine color is another way of determining if you have rehydrated. Dark urine means that it is too concentrated and you need to consume more fluid.

- Fluids used should be cool (about fifty to seventy degrees Fahrenheit) to help lower body temperature and empty them from the stomach rapidly.

- Avoid beverages containing alcohol, because their diuretic effect can lead to dehydration. (Caffeinated beverages are okay; they are not a strong enough diuretic to cause dehydration.)

- Individual response to caffeine-containing drinks varies; those who normally ingest caffeine may tolerate it better, while others may experience upset stomach and/or jittery muscles that can impede performance. Carbonated beverages may cause gastrointestinal discomfort.

- Water is generally a satisfactory choice. Sports drinks can be used if they contain no more than 8 percent carbohydrate and a small number of electrolytes. Sports drinks can be beneficial for activities lasting about sixty minutes or more.

- Weight should return to within two pounds of beginning weight before resuming activity.

Electrolytes can generally be replenished during the next meal. During long, strenuous bouts of activity in the heat, however (particularly those lasting longer than three hours), electrolytes can be lost in amounts sufficient to cause physiological problems. Fluids with small amounts of electrolytes (e.g., most sports drinks) can be advantageous under these circumstances.

The 6 Percent Solution

When exercising or competing in events of more than sixty minutes, particularly if they are high-intensity, you may want to consider a sports drink. Specially formulated sports drinks can aid your performance by providing energy in the form of carbohydrate. They can also replenish the electrolytes that we lose from our bodies via sweat. As with many things, more is not necessarily better. Look for sports drinks that provide nominal amounts of carbohydrate—about 6 percent. The greater the carbohydrate content above 6 percent, the higher the risk of gastrointestinal upset. (Although individuals differ in tolerance, carbohydrate content up to 8 percent may be okay.) To determine if a drink meets the "6 percent solution," be a Sherlock and sleuth it out. Here's how:

1. Convert ounces to milliliters (ml). If the label lists a serving as eight ounces, multiply by thirty (the approximate number of ml in one ounce) to determine the ml of fluid in one serving. ($8 \times 30 = 240$ ml)

2. Divide the grams (g) of carbohydrate (CHO) listed for a serving by the number of ml in a serving. For example, if there are fourteen grams listed for a serving, then divide fourteen by the number of ml of fluid in a serving.

So, if you have a drink and its serving size is listed as eight ounces, with fourteen grams of CHO, does this meet the 6 percent solution? Let's see:

8 ounces × 30 ml per ounce = 240 ml

14 g CHO/240 ml = .058 (rounded off to 6 percent)

Okay, down the hatch! Your drink meets the carb requirement for hydration during activity.

But if you don't have a sports drink handy, don't worry. Grab some 100 percent fruit juice and dilute it 50/50 with water. You'll have your own homemade 6 percent-solution sports drink!

CHAPTER THIRTEEN:

How to Lose Weight ...
and Not Find It Again!

ONLY 20–30 PERCENT OF PEOPLE who lose weight are successful in maintaining 5–10 percent of lost weight. Contributors to weight gain are poor portion control, sugar-sweetened beverage consumption, more meals eaten outside of the home, lack of physical activity, calorie overconsumption, and stress. Today's high-tech, energy-saving devices, coupled with a plethora of available food and beverage, is the perfect storm for gaining weight and keeping it.

There are lots of factors that make it easy to gain weight, difficult to lose it, and even harder to keep it off. Conversely—in the spirit of optimism or looking at it from the "glass half full" perspective—this means there are lots of things we can do to reverse this!

This is good, because everyone is different, and what may work for one person may not for another. There is no one correct way to approach weight management. I hope you can find things within this chapter that resonate with you and will help you in your quest to achieve and maintain a healthy weight.

Begin by Setting Realistic Goals

The first thing you want to do is set goals that are realistic, specific, measurable, and time-sensitive. Doing this will enable you to make gradual changes in your lifestyle that will last. You didn't gain your excess weight overnight, so you shouldn't try to lose it all at once. If you set unrealistic goals, you may wind up discouraged and quit. Losing a pound or two a week is reasonable, and the pounds lost add up fast.

Continue motivating yourself with small successes. Specific actions that can be measured will allow you to do this. For example, start out with a goal of replacing a regular soda each day with a glass of water (possibly with no- or low-calorie flavoring). Determine that you'll do this for a week or two and then add another modest goal to reach. (See chapter 1 for specific strategies on how to accomplish this.) Before you know it, you'll have created a healthy diet and lifestyle!

Control Your Environment

We all know that things such as "willpower" and "self-discipline" are much easier to refer to than to have. Therefore, in an effort to avoid having to rely on these traits, we should lead ourselves away from temptation as much as possible. And with a bit of forethought and planning, we can make this possible.

We can create an environment that allows us the opportunity to make healthy lifestyle choices with the least effort. Next to our place of work, we spend most of our waking hours at home, and as it happens, this is the place in which we can exert the most control. So, if we have a problem resisting a chocolate bar's beckoning call, we shouldn't bring them home ("out of sight, out of mind," or at least "out of reach!").

Often, fruit and vegetables are kept hidden in a bottom drawer of the refrigerator. The only time we notice them is when we're doing our occasional purge of the fridge for spoiled foods that have long been neglected. It makes you wonder if our garbage containers aren't eating healthier than we are! Keeping fruit and veggies more accessible and noticeable will greatly increase the probability that we'll eat them when having a snack attack, rather than that fat- and sugar-loaded cake, pie, or candy.

When we do eat at home, we should beware of distractions. We tend to eat more while watching TV, working on the computer, playing games, etc., because we are distracted and lose touch with our bodies' signals telling us we're full. We also may eat more to get satisfied, because we haven't really savored the food we've been eating. Whenever possible, meals and snacks should be eaten mindfully, without distraction, with the exception of good family conversation around the dinner table.

Most of us (myself included) do at times eat while watching television, working on the computer, or doing other types of things that tend to distract us. When I'm snacking while watching my favorite show at night, I take precautions to avoid unconsciously overeating. I like to snack on popcorn, which is a whole grain and a pretty good choice, as long as I don't douse it with butter and salt. I buy microwaveable 100-calorie bags. Then, no matter how distracted I am, I can't consume more than 100 calories. If I'm snacking on dark chocolate, I get two or three squares (a serving or less) and put the remainder of the bar away. In order to make it last, I take small bites and savor each by allowing it to melt in my mouth. Doing this enables me to get satisfaction from the chocolate that lasts throughout my television show.

If we find ourselves in circumstances where we can't exert control over our environment, such as eating away from home, then we need to plan for and scout out environments that are more health friendly. This could mean checking out which restaurants offer healthy, nutritious options prior to going out to lunch with colleagues. Most restaurants have their menus on their websites, as well as nutrition information. Don't go into a fast food burger place if you're an easy mark for a bacon cheese-burger and fries. Find a place that emphasizes healthier bites and doesn't hit you with the aroma of fries as soon as you enter. You could also choose to eat at a restaurant within walking distance of your job, so as to fit in some physical activity.

Get together with like-minded colleagues at work, and lobby for healthy choices in the vending machines, or having mini bagels and low-fat yogurt with water at meetings instead of just donuts, pastries, and soda. Have healthy potlucks, team fitness competitions, and/or start a break-time walking group and walk around the building, either inside or outside (weather permitting).

Eat Bulky

Research shows that, over the course of a day or two, a person will eat about the same weight (bulk) of food. Therefore, eating foods that have a lot of bulk but are low in calories will help you manage your weight.

Water and fiber provide weight to food that makes you feel full with fewer calories. So, eating plenty of nutrient-dense, low-calorie foods with large amounts of water and fiber, such as fruits, vegetables, brothy soups, low-fat milk, and cooked whole grains will fill you up before you con-sume too many calories. Since you eat plenty of food and are satiated, you are more prone to do this long term. This is in contrast to foods such as potato chips (bet you can't eat just one!) and glazed donuts that are high in calories but low in weight, allowing you to eat a bunch, along with loads of calories!

Where are the calories?

- Fat = nine calories per gram weight
- Alcohol = seven calories per gram weight
- Protein = four calories per gram weight
- Carbohydrate = four calories per gram weight
- Fiber = two calories per gram weight
- Water = zero calories per gram weight

Where's the Fiber?

- Fruits and vegetables (especially the skin)
- Whole grains (slice of bread should have at least two grams fiber per slice, and cereal at least three grams per serving)
- Brown rice and whole wheat pasta
- Dried beans and peas

Other Strategies

- Write down what you eat and drink, then enter it into a program to analyze it (many free smartphone apps will allow you to do this).
- Weigh regularly and record it (this helps you know if you are getting off track with your weight and motivates you to make changes before it gets out of hand).
- Check out the restaurant menu before going to determine if it has healthy, low-calorie choices.
- When dishing out food at home, use a smaller plate. This makes it appear you are getting enough food, and you are less likely to overeat. You can always get seconds if you're still hungry.
- Eat more frequently (e.g., three meals and a healthy snack or two per day).
- Eat slowly and savor your food; it takes your stomach about twenty minutes to tell your brain you are full.

- Eat sufficient amounts of lean protein at each meal, as it makes you feel full longer (also, protein is harder to digest, so you use more calories to do so).
- Practice portion control, as studies show people eat more when given bigger portions (portions are what we, or restaurants, give us, not USDA serving sizes; portions have tended to increase over time).
  - Read labels carefully to determine the suggested serving size and how many calories they contain.
  - Get a feel for the USDA recommended serving size by measuring out foods at home until you are familiar with them.
- Beware of what may be false hunger signals, such as
  - The craving or urge to eat a certain food.
  - Feeling emotional: angry, lonely, or sad.
  - Being bored or stressed.
  - Thirst—it is sometimes misinterpreted as hunger. Try drinking water or another noncaloric beverage, and then see if you still feel hungry.

Stay within Your Budget!

Weight loss and gain are mainly determined by a simple formula—calories in versus calories out. To lose weight, you need to create a calorie deficit by burning more than you consume. Do the opposite and you gain weight. To maintain a healthy weight, you need them to be balanced.

Think of weight control and nutrients in the same way you would think of your financial budget. Calories expended through activity represent money you earn and can spend, and calories consumed are money you have spent. You should first use your money earned to pay your bills—

to get the nutrients you need for health—while not spending more money (calories) than you earn. Spending (consuming) more calories than you earn (e.g., burning through physical activity) has consequences (gaining weight) just as it does to spend more money than you have (going into debt). And just as if you would confer with a CPA about your more complex financials, any questions you have regarding nutrition issues should be addressed to a registered dietitian.

Maintaining Weight Loss—Keep It Going for Life

Lifestyle choices leading to weight management and health must remain at the forefront of your consciousness and be part of a lifetime journey to maintain success. And think about how much time and energy people spend on dieting and related activities. If as much time, effort, and thought were devoted to making healthy lifestyle choices, success would be much more commonplace. Like anything else, once you've done it for a while and it is habitual and incorporated into your life, it is not seen as so much extra effort. And think about it: if you lose your health, the rest of the things in your life become moot anyway!

Genetics, or other circumstances beyond someone's control, may make it difficult for many to lose weight. If this is the case, adhering to a healthy lifestyle will, at the very least, ensure that you are in a better state of health. Also, other options are becoming more available, such as medications, surgery, and surgical devices. Having been around for some time now, many of these options have become safer and more successful than in the past. Consult with your doctor to see what might be best for you.

Every Little Bit Helps

Even small amounts of weight loss can have significant health benefits—especially for diabetes, heart disease, and other health problems affected or caused by weight. We should be concerned not only about living longer but about how we live those extra years. We want those years to be healthy, good-quality ones!

CHAPTER FOURTEEN:

How Sweet It Is ... or Not?

MANY OF MY PATIENTS HAVE RESERVATIONS about using artificial sweeteners. This is not surprising, given the controversy regarding how they may affect our health. While most studies have found them to be safe, anecdotal evidence from individuals indicates they may cause headaches or other minor side effects in some people.

I have had several patients that, while trying to eat healthier and lose weight, were adding many calories from sugar because they had heard bad things about artificial sweeteners. Sugar adds calories without nutrients, can cause dental caries (cavities), and is associated with a higher risk of heart disease. Even if all the negatives about low- and no-calorie sweeteners were true, they still wouldn't be as bad for you as added sugars appear to be. Personally, I use sweeteners made from stevia. It is the most natural no-calorie sweetener currently on the market.

There has been much debate as to whether food and beverages made with artificial sweeteners actually help weight loss and maintenance or whether they hinder it. One theory suggests that the intense sweetness of diet beverages may entice the taste buds and cause people to seek out and consume more calories from sweet foods and beverages. This is merely conjecture, however, because there is currently little scientific evidence to confirm this. The well-controlled studies done so far actually show that using artificial sweeteners in place of sugar leads to more weight loss. The fear of artificial sweeteners causing cancer has also been shown to be scientifically unfounded thus far.

Future studies may either confirm or refute these conflicting beliefs and theories. We'll just have to wait and see. In the meantime, artificial sweeteners may be a good alternative for sugar, especially given the problems sugar can cause for our health.

Most health organizations and health professionals consider artificial sweeteners to be an acceptable tool that can be used to keep blood sugar from spiking. They have been a very helpful tool for diabetics, who must keep their blood sugar under control to avoid health complications. Many also depend on the use of noncaloric sweeteners for weight management, replacing the calories in foods and beverages otherwise laden with sugar.

If a sugar substitute has caused you problems in the past, you might try other types. The FDA has approved a number of artificial sweeteners as safe for use, based on existing scientific evidence. This includes calorie-free sweeteners that are more naturally derived from plants, such as stevia and monk fruit. Most of the plant-derived substitutes are made with all-natural ingredients. To ensure this is the case, read the ingredients label when shopping for them.

So far, no- and low-calorie sweeteners have been found to be our best alternative to sugar. Good commonsense evaluation of new products is prudent. It seems that after decades of studies, however, sugar alternatives appear to be a safe, useful alternative to the added sugars in our diets.

CHAPTER FIFTEEN:

Is Vegetarian the Healthier Way to Go?

ARE VEGETARIAN DIETS HEALTHIER than those that include meat? I am often asked this question, and the answer is simply, "Yes and no."

I'm not waffling with my answer—or maybe I am, a little. I mean to point out that many diets can be healthy, both meat-eating and vegetarian, but it takes careful planning to consume a variety of foods and beverages that will provide all the nutrients necessary for good health. Since the vegetarian diet omits certain animal-based foods and beverages, a little more care and planning is warranted.

How much more care and planning? It depends on what type of vegetarian diet you choose to follow. And there are plenty! Vegetarian types include (in descending order from liberal to strict) the following:

- Flexitarian: a bit more liberal about it and will occasionally eat meat, poultry, fish, and seafood.
- Pollotarian: eat poultry, such as chicken and turkey, but avoid red meat, fish, and seafood.
- Pescatarian: will avoid meat and poultry but eat fish and seafood.

- Lacto-ovo-vegetarian: avoid all types of meat, fish and seafood but eat eggs and dairy.
- Lacto-vegetarian: eat dairy but avoid eggs and all types of meat, fish, and seafood.
- Ovo-vegetarian: do not eat poultry, red meat, fish, seafood, or dairy but will eat eggs.
- Vegan: avoid all animal products, including anything derived from animals (e.g., eggs, dairy).

A plant-based diet can be a nutritious way to eat. After all, you have nutritious fruits, vegetables, grains, legumes, and nuts on the menu. Since most of our diets are pretty sparse in the area of plant foods, we don't get enough of the healthy, chronic-disease-fighting nutrients provided with them. A vegetarian diet can ensure that we get enough of these plant-based treasures.

So, to be sure that we get the "best of both worlds"—a healthy vegetarian diet, as well as all the nutrients we require—there are certain nutritional considerations that must be taken into account:

- Don't worry so much about complimentary protein to get all your essential amino acids. Eating a variety of vegetables and whole grains will help ensure that you're getting adequate amounts of high-quality protein. And as long as you consume them the same day—not necessarily at the same meal, as once thought—that's fine.
- Dairy, of course, is a good source of calcium and vitamin D. If you are a vegan, however, look for calcium-fortified foods and beverages, such as orange juice, soy milk, and tofu made with calcium. Some vegetables have small to moderate amounts of calcium, such as broccoli, kale, collard/turnip/mustard greens and bok choy.

- Vitamin D food sources, other than dairy, include cold-water fish (e.g. salmon, swordfish, tuna, mackerel, and sardines), fortified margarines, egg yolks, and beef liver. Beef liver is likely out if you are vegetarian, and if you are a strict vegan, and don't eat fish or eggs, you may need to consider a vitamin D supplement.

- Vitamin B_{12} is found only in animal products, so look for foods fortified with B_{12} or take a B_{12} supplement. Better yet, consider taking a daily multiple vitamin / mineral supplement to get your B_{12} plus the recommended daily amounts of other vitamins and minerals.

- Plants contain substances that can inhibit zinc absorption. Therefore, vegetarians need to consume about 50 percent more zinc than nonvegetarians. Sources of zinc include soybeans and soymilk, beans, nuts, dairy, whole grain, and fortified products such as breakfast cereals, mushrooms, and wheat germ.

- Meat provides the most absorbable form of iron. Therefore, meat abstainers should be sure to eat plenty of iron-rich plant foods— fortified breakfast cereals and breads, soy-based foods, dried fruit, nuts, and beans. Consuming a vitamin C source enhances absorption of iron from nonmeat sources. Some vitamin C sources include broccoli, bell peppers, tomatoes, citrus fruit, watermelon, kiwi fruit, berries, and salad greens. Also, cooking in an iron skillet increases the iron content of the food being cooked. The iron from the pan leaches into the food, especially if it's an acidic food such as tomato sauce. Don't drink tea or coffee or consume high-calcium foods or beverages with iron-containing foods, as they can block the absorption of iron. Be sure to get your iron status checked by your doctor regularly, especially in the case of a child who is still growing or a premenopausal or pregnant woman.

Take high-dosage iron supplements only if they are prescribed by your doctor.

All vegetarian diets, especially the vegan diet, have health advantages, which include lower dietary intakes of saturated fat and cholesterol and higher intakes of fiber and many nutrients that we often do not get enough of, such as vitamins A and C. Plants also have an abundance of phytonutrients, substances that lower our risk of contracting chronic diseases like heart disease, diabetes, and many types of cancer. A vegetarian diet is also associated with lower body weight.

Good nutrition takes planning. If you are a vegetarian, it may take a bit more planning to ensure you're getting what you need. This is becoming easier, though. More people are choosing to go vegetarian, and so mainstream markets are now carrying most of the newly formulated food and beverage products that cater to this demand. This makes it easier to successfully navigate a vegetarian diet while getting the nutrition your body needs.

So, if you feel inclined, go for it! When done right, a vegetarian diet can be a healthy one, considering all the plant foods you'll be eating!

CHAPTER SIXTEEN:

Nutrition and Activity Needs of Older Adults

OLDER ADULTS HAVE MORE LIFE EXPERIENCES, knowledge, patience, and wisdom than younger people do. They have learned from their mistakes and so are less likely to duplicate them. There are good reasons to not wish to be a teenager again!

But older adults undergo various physiological and social changes that can have a deleterious effect on their health. Seniors are generally unable to efficiently absorb and utilize many of the vitamins and minerals their bodies need. If they are retired, they may lack routine in their lives, including when to eat. If they are widowed and living by themselves, they may forget to prepare and eat a meal for just themselves. This is why many seniors are at risk for nutritional deficiencies.

Older adults are often less active. If they no longer work, they tend to be more sedentary in their lifestyles. They no longer get up, travel to a job, work, and socialize with colleagues. Also, physical infirmity may limit mobility and make regular physical activity more difficult. Thus, the health benefits from regular physical activity become more limited as one ages.

Seniors don't need to accept an unhealthy state in their golden years, however. They just need to be aware of the specific needs of older adults and be vigilant about living a lifestyle that addresses these needs. Let's look at some of the ways in which they may overcome some of the obstacles to healthy aging.

Fluid Needs

Adequate water consumption reduces stress on kidney function, which tends to decline with age. Try to drink at least six to eight glasses of water, juice, milk, and coffee or tea every day (more under certain circumstances, such as being physically active in the heat). Don't wait until you're thirsty, as the ability to detect thirst declines as we age.

Eat plenty of fruits and vegetables. Produce is mostly water, so it will provide extra hydration. This is a bonus health benefit they provide, in addition to antioxidants that can lower the risk of chronic diseases. Soups, puddings, and yogurt are examples of other foods that can provide a significant amount of fluid that the body requires.

Reduced Calories

As we age, our metabolism slows, and we tend to be less active, so we need to consume fewer calories to maintain a healthy weight. This means we must choose our diets more carefully to get the nutrients we need. Nutrient-dense foods, such as fruits and vegetables, can fit this bill.

But be careful to consume enough food via regular meals and snacks. Sufficient calories must be consumed to meet energy needs. Too few calories mean that body protein will be broken down and used for energy instead of other crucial physiological needs—hormones, enzymes, cell rebuilding, muscle, etc. Seniors have a higher rate of muscle loss in general, making it even more crucial that they get enough calories to avoid more muscle breakdown.

Extra Protein

Our bodies need a certain amount of protein for cell replacement, enzymes, hormones, fluid balance, acid-base regulation, transport substances, antibodies, wound healing, immunity, and energy. The recommended amount for healthy adults is 0.8 grams per kilogram of body weight. Since we are less active and have less of an appetite as we age, we generally consume fewer calories and, thus, less protein. Therefore, we must intake protein at a higher ratio—at least 1.0 grams per kilogram of body weight, unless a condition (such as kidney disease) warrants a smaller amount. Divide your weight in pounds by 2.2, and you'll get your weight in kilograms. Your weight in kilograms is the same as the number of grams of protein you should consume daily. For example, if you are 165 pounds, divide that by 2.2 and you get 75. Therefore, your weight is seventy-five kilograms and you should consume at least seventy-five grams of protein each day.

Good sources of high-quality protein are lean meat, poultry, seafood, and eggs. Good plant-based sources of protein are dried beans and peas, nuts and nut butters, soybean products, and mixtures of whole grains and vegetables. Mixtures of beans and grains, and vegetables and grains, eaten throughout the day, will provide all the essential amino acids for high-quality protein.

Vitamin D and Calcium

We lose bone density as we get older, particularly women after menopause. Vitamin D helps our bodies absorb calcium to maintain the structural integrity of our bones and teeth. As we age, we tend to be outside less often, and when we are outside our bodies cannot make vitamin D from sunlight as efficiently as when we were younger. Between the ages of fifty and seventy, we need at least 600 IUs (International Units) of vitamin D each day (800 IUs after age seventy). Food sources for vitamin D are fatty fish, fish liver oils, fortified milk and milk products, cereals, and other fortified foods and beverages.

Calcium, the most abundant mineral in the body, is important for our health and well-being. In addition to creating strong bones and teeth, it aids in muscle contraction, blood pressure, nerve transmission, and many other bodily functions. Good sources of calcium are low-fat dairy products, canned fish with bones (e.g., sardines), and calcium-fortified foods and beverages. Also, weight-bearing exercises (walking, aerobics, strength training) help strengthen bones.

Vitamin B$_{12}$

As we age, our stomachs become less acidic. Since the substance in our bodies that extracts B$_{12}$ from food needs an acidic environment, B$_{12}$ is not obtained from food as readily as when we were younger. We need 2.4 mcg (micrograms) per day. Food sources include meat, fish, poultry, milk, and fortified cereals. Since we lose some of our capacity to absorb this vitamin from food as we age, we may need to get the supplement form from fortified foods and vitamin supplements.

Vitamin B$_6$

Some vitamin B$_6$ functions include helping build red blood cells, forming proteins, and maintaining brain and nervous system operation. Men need 1.7 mg (milligrams) and women 1.5 mg daily. Vitamin B6 food sources are whole grains, organ meats, nuts, bananas, potatoes, fish, poultry, avocado, legumes, and fortified soy-based meat substitutes.

Fiber

Adequate fiber, along with adequate fluid intake, helps maintain normal bowel function and lowers the risk of some diseases. Eat plenty of fruits, vegetables, whole grains, and legumes. You should consume at least fourteen grams of fiber for every 1,000 calories, as a rule of thumb. This means most people should have in the area of twenty-five to thirty grams per day. When first increasing fiber intake, be sure to drink plenty of fluids to avoid intestinal gas and bloating.

Multiple Vitamin / Mineral Supplement

Taking a supplement from a reputable company that contains no more than the approximate recommended daily allowance for most nutrients is a good way to ensure you will not be deficient. Look for the symbols with USP (United States Pharmacopeia) or CL (ConsumerLabs.com) on the container. This means the supplement has been tested by an independent laboratory and meets the stringent criteria set for the manufacturing of dietary supplements. Store brands often have the same or similar ingredients at a significant reduction in price. If you buy from a reputable store brand, you increase the chance that you are getting a quality product, even if it is not tested by an independent laboratory.

Be sure to inform your doctor of any supplements you are taking to be sure they don't interact with medications that you may be taking or health conditions for which you are being treated.

Muscle Loss

Beginning in our mid- to late twenties, we lose approximately 2 percent of our muscle mass each decade. By the time we reach our fifties and sixties, we are at risk of sarcopenia, severe loss of muscle that limits an individual's mobility and independence.

Exercise can counter much of the loss of muscle tissue from aging. Incorporate aerobic exercise with strength training. Aerobic exercise can be walking, swimming, water aerobics, dancing, gardening, bike riding, or other moderate activities that increase endurance. Strength training builds and maintains muscle, so that you can maintain the strength necessary to avoid falls and live independently.

Prior to beginning an exercise program, see your doctor to determine any limitations you may have. Kick your program off by seeing a fitness professional or physical therapist to make sure you are doing exercises correctly and in a way that will not injure you.

Getting older is inevitable, but becoming less healthy is not. It may take a bit more effort, but the quality of life that results is certainly worth it. So bring on that bucket list!

CHAPTER SEVENTEEN:

Information on Individual Foods and Beverages

Introduction

Whether you want to avoid or mitigate a chronic disease, retard the aging process, or just look better, consuming a variety of the foods and beverages contained in this chapter should be just what the doctor ordered.

Foodstuffs are made up of thousands of bioactive substances that positively affect health. Some are traditional nutrients, such as vitamins, minerals, and fiber. Others are beneficial compounds called phytochemicals that are being discovered by nutritional scientists.

Phytochemicals ("phyto" being Greek for plant) are substances in plants that protect them from disease and predators. When we eat plants, we also gain this disease-fighting protection (which is why phytochemicals are often referred to as phytonutrients). Studies have indicated that these substances act in tandem to achieve optimal benefits. Also, we have only scratched the surface in regard to discovering all of these types of substances that exist in food. Given that, it is important to obtain these nutrients from food, not supplements. This is why nutrition experts recommend eating a diet that is varied and plant based.

Most phytochemical compounds are actually pigments, which is where fruits and vegetables get their colorful appearances. This is why registered dietitians and nutrition education literature will sometimes declare the importance of including a rainbow of colors in your eating plan.

Fruits and Vegetables

(serving size = ½ cup, one cup of raw leafy greens,
four ounces of 100 percent juice)

- Eat a variety of fruits and vegetables, as each type offers different amounts and varieties of the thousands of substances we're finding in plant foods, called phytochemicals or phytonutrients. Many studies linking fruit and vegetable consumption to lower risk of disease have associated the effect with eating a variety of fruits and vegetables.

- The most inexpensive way to purchase fruits and vegetables is to buy them canned, frozen, or in season. Canned fruits and vegetables are almost as nutritious as fresh ones, and frozen varieties are just as nutritious if not more so. Frozen fruits and vegetables are flash-frozen immediately after being picked. This deactivates enzymes that would degrade the nutrients, keeping the produce as nutritious as if you ate it at the farm!

Apples

(serving size = one medium apple or ½ cup)

- There are about 7,500 varieties of apples grown throughout the world, although there are fewer than ten popular varieties commonly sold in the United States. Red Delicious is the variety richest in phenolic compounds, nontraditional nutrients that provide many of apples' health benefits. Be sure to eat the whole apple, as its health-providing nutrients are found in both the meat and skin.

- Apples, like many other fruits, produce a natural wax coating to prevent water loss. This prevents shriveling and weight loss of the fruit. After harvesting, apples are washed to remove dust and chemical residues. This removes about half of the natural wax, which is replaced by a coating of artificial wax (only about one to two drops per fruit to produce a microscopic covering). This allows apples to maintain their quality and attractiveness. Although the wax is safe to consume, it is recommended that you wash apples, as well as other fruit, with cool tap water without soap or detergent just before eating. Drying them with a clean cloth towel or paper towel may further reduce any bacteria or pesticide residue that may be present.

- Chopped apples added to pancakes or salads provide great taste, crunch, fiber, and added nutrients.

Avocados
(serving size = 1/3 of medium-sized fruit or about 50 grams)

- Often mistaken for a vegetable, the much-loved avocado is actually a fruit. The two most popular types are Florida and Hass (mainly from California) avocados. Florida avocados have a fruity taste and are lower in fat, while the Hass avocados have a nutty, buttery flavor.

- Avocados are high in monounsaturated fat, the kind that has been shown to have health benefits. There is evidence from at least one well-done study that indicates they may reduce your risk of heart disease by lowering your total and LDL (bad) cholesterol.

- After cutting into an avocado, rub lemon juice on the surface of the portion you wish to save, as this will keep it from turning brown.

Bananas

(serving size = one medium banana or ½ cup)

- Bananas are composed of three sugars—sucrose, fructose and glucose—along with a good dose of fiber. Together they provide plenty of sustained carbohydrate energy for fueling activity. This is why so many athletes consume bananas before, during, and after long training sessions or competitions.

- Eat bananas that are not too ripe, just slightly green at the tip, to receive the maximum health benefits.

- Bananas are nice and soft, and can be added to almost anything, such as smoothies, pancake or waffle batter or baked items. Try peeling one, freezing it, then putting it in a food blender for a consistency that is similar to ice cream. Add a little syrup and some nuts and you have a healthy sundae!

Beans and Peas, Dried

(serving size = ½ cup)

- All dried beans and peas, except lentils and split peas, require soaking in water for rehydration. About three cups of water are needed for each cup of dried beans. Beans should soak overnight, be rinsed in clean water, then covered in water and cooked in a stock pot. (Soaking will also help eliminate hard-to-digest sugars responsible for the mild discomfort associated with bean ingestion.)

- Use beans as an inexpensive meat alternative in chili, casseroles, and other mealtime dishes. Beans are high in protein and a good source of iron, fiber, and folate.

Berries

(serving size = ½ cup)

- Antioxidants in berries, called flavonoids, can protect cells from many of the ravages of aging. Vitamin C, a strong antioxidant, is also found in berries in plentiful supply. As with other types of foods, eating a variety of berries will help ensure you are getting all of the different types of phytonutrients that provide health benefits.

- **Blackberries** are high in ellagic acid, vitamin C, and fiber, substances that may lower cancer risk. They have one of the highest antioxidant levels of any fruit. They are high in folate and also have antiviral and antibacterial properties. Do not wash blackberries until you are ready to use them, as they can easily become waterlogged. They can be refrigerated for up to two days or frozen for up to nine months.

- **Blueberries** are high in fiber and have the highest antioxidant properties of any fruit—but eating them with milk may impair the antioxidant properties. In a memory study, only one half-cup serving of blueberries or two half-cup servings of strawberries each week were needed to reap the benefits. Not having a strong, distinctive taste, blueberries blend well with almost any type of foodstuff. Blueberry pancakes, anyone? Also, make a triple berry pie (blueberries, strawberries, and raspberries) with graham cracker crust as a healthy, refreshing summer desert. Wild blueberries, ubiquitous in the state of Maine, are small in size but tasty. So if you happen upon a diner while traveling in Maine, definitely order the blueberry pie—you won't regret it!

- **Fiber-rich** cranberries are one of only three major fruits native to North America, along with blueberries and Concord grapes. Fresh cranberries are generally available in the cooler months of September to December, while the juices and sauce are available year-round in grocery stores. For a Thanksgiving treat, or a healthy additional to any meal, grind cranberries in a food processor with other fruit, such as apples, oranges, or dried apricots.

- **Raspberries** and blackberries are both cane berries, growing on woody canes or stems rather than bushes. Raspberries are highest in fiber among the berries, with a whopping eight grams per cup! Raspberries mold easily, so do not wash them until they're ready to use. They last only a couple of days in the refrigerator, so when you purchase raspberries, be prepared to use them! Store them uncovered in the refrigerator as soon as possible after purchasing. If fresh raspberries aren't available, try to get your hands on the freeze-dried berries; they are just as nutritious and will last longer. They are great for pies and salads for topping cereals or as a smoothie ingredient.

- **Strawberries** have about three times the vitamin C of the next highest berry and are tied with blackberries for providing the most folate per cup. These beautiful red, heart-shaped fruits are somewhat of an aberration, though, in that their seeds are on the outside rather than the inside. What was Mother Nature thinking? No matter; strawberries are delicious and good for you, so, kudos to you, Mother Nature! Strawberries have a strong fragrance. If you can't smell them, don't buy them, as they do not continue to ripen after harvesting. Serve them at room temperature for best taste. Use strawberries to spice up salads, sweeten hot cereals, or add a nutritional punch to smoothies.

Brazil Nuts
(serving size = one ounce)

- Brazil nuts are one of the few foods that provide significant amounts of selenium. Eating just a couple of them daily provides enough to meet daily selenium requirements and confer the associated health benefits.

- Do not eat more than a few Brazil nuts daily, and avoid taking large doses of selenium supplements, as too much of it can be toxic.

Carrots
(serving size = ½ cup)

- Carotenoids provide much of the health benefits of carrots. They are best absorbed by chopping and cooking carrots in oil to release the carotenoids from the cell membranes.

- Steam carrots and add a bit of olive oil and pepper for taste. The heat and oil will allow maximum absorption of the carrot phytonutrients. Cutting the carrots after cooking rather than before will preserve more of the nutrients.

Celery
(serving size = ½ cup)

- Although considered by most to not be very nutritious, this stalky veggie of Mediterranean origin contains phytochemicals (nontraditional nutrients found in plants) that can be very beneficial to our health. It is also a good source of potassium, folate, fiber, molybdenum, manganese, and vitamin B_6.

- Yes, the old "ants on a log" is a great snack, particularly for kids. In addition to the celery's phytonutrients, peanut butter is a good source of protein and healthy monounsaturated fat, while raisins pack their own nutritional punch.

Cherries

(serving size = ½ cup, ¼ cup dried)

- Cherries have been found to have nutrients with strong anti-inflammatory power. Since inflammation is associated with so many disease states, cherries may play an important role in a healthy diet.

- For those who don't like tart tastes but have tart cherries, make a pie with sweetener or remove the pits and mix with ice cream, smoothies, etc.

Chocolate, Dark

(serving size = one ounce)

- Cacao beans are not actually beans but seeds from the fruit of the cacao tree. Natural cacao contains hundreds of different nutrients that may be beneficial, many of which are just now being discovered.

- Doses used in health studies vary widely, but a moderate portion size of chocolate is considered to be about one ounce. Remember, although it has health benefits, it is high in fat, saturated fat, and calories. Eating too much of it can undo its health benefits.

- There are no FDA standards of identity for dark chocolate. Therefore, it is best to look for dark chocolate bars that have the percent cacao listed. Choose a bar with at least 70 percent cacao to get an appreciable amount of flavonoids for health benefits.

- To avoid overindulging, take a square or two and nibble small bites. Rather than immediately chewing and swallowing, savor each bite by letting it melt in your mouth. This will satisfy your taste buds with minimal calorie intake.

Citrus Fruit

(serving size = ½ cup, four ounces 100 percent juice)

- When peeling a citrus fruit, don't be too careful about taking off the white under peel, as it has been found to contain nutrients beneficial to health—such as hesperidin for lowering blood pressure and cholesterol.

- Have half a grapefruit or some orange slices with your cereal. The vitamin C from the fruit will increase the absorption of the iron in the cereal.

Coffee

(serving size = six to eight ounces)

- If you're not currently a java junkie, health authorities advise not to begin drinking coffee for health benefits, but rather to eat plenty of plant foods, such as fruits and vegetables. High amounts of caffeine in pregnancy may increase the risk of miscarriage and may exacerbate reflux disease (severe indigestion/heartburn). Brewing coffee using the French press method does not filter out many of the oils that can affect the liver, raising LDL cholesterol (the unhealthy kind).

- Be careful about the type of coffee you get and what you put in it. Adding sugar, syrups, and cream can cancel out any health benefits, and some specialty coffees can pack up to 500 calories or more, leading to weight gain. Some studies found that both regular and decaf coffee lowered the risk of certain diseases, especially type 2 diabetes, indicating that coffee contains substances other than caffeine that are responsible for the benefits.

- Use artificial sweetener, cinnamon, and skim milk as add-ins to your java juice, as these are limited in calories and other negatives that many coffee flavorings contain.

Cruciferous Vegetables

(serving size = ½ cup, one cup raw cabbage leaves)

- Studies indicate that health benefits may be derived from eating just one serving per day of cruciferous vegetables. However, some studies also indicate that consuming more may increase these benefits. To get the most benefit, eat your crucifers raw.

- Native to the Mediterranean, **arugula** was considered by ancient Romans and Egyptians to be an aphrodisiac. It is low in calories and very nutritious. It's a source of vitamins A, C, and K and folate, calcium, fiber, and potassium. Choose dark greens leaves and avoid leaves that are yellowing. Remove the tough stems before cleaning. As with mustard greens and watercress, add arugula to salads for a peppery flavoring. Mix with other greens to tone down its potent flavor. If cooking arugula, do so only for a few seconds, or its peppery flavor will dissipate.

- High in vitamins A and C, **bok choy** is a popular vegetable in Chinese and Southeast Asian cooking. Leafy green and cruciferous, it is closely related to cabbage and provides numerous health benefits for only about thirteen calories per serving. It can be used in salads, sandwiches, and stir fries. To maintain bok choy's original flavor and preserve nutrients, the best cooking method is steaming.

- Sulforaphane is the substance that provides much of **broccoli**'s nutrient punch. It can be degraded by heat, so that eating broccoli raw will give you the most health benefits. Tests revealed that the amount of sulforaphane absorbed was ten times higher for raw than for cooked broccoli. To get your child to eat broccoli or cauliflower florets, mix them with spaghetti sauce. They have the shape and texture of meatballs but are hidden by the sauce! Also, chop up the florets and include them as one of the ingredients in an omelet. Broccoli florets are great eaten raw with low-fat dip or dispersed throughout a salad. Although healthiest raw, lightly steamed is the next best way to prepare broccoli. It allows it to keep its crunch without cooking out much of the nutritious phytonutrients. If preparing for only one to four people, inexpensive, microwavable plastic steamers can be found online. Larger ones are also available for bigger families.

- **Broccoli rabe**—high in vitamins A, C, and K and potassium—is actually more closely related to the turnip than to broccoli. It can be steamed, sautéed, blanched, boiled, or stir-fried. When using the stems, cook them for about two minutes before adding the leaves, and then cook for another one to two minutes. Add to soups and casseroles or stir-fry them with other veggies and meats.

- **Brussels sprouts** are high in vitamins A, C, and K and folate, and fiber. They are members of the cabbage family, and actually appear to be miniature cabbages. Yes, Brussels sprouts are very popular in Brussels, Belgium, and may have originated there. Steaming, roasting, microwaving, and stir-frying are the best ways to cook Brussels sprouts, as boiling can result in significant loss of many of their nutrients.

- **Cabbage** comes in various shades of green as well as red and purple. Although there are hundreds of varieties, the most popular in the United States are green cabbage and bok choy. Cabbage is rich in nutrients, including beta-carotene, vitamin C, and fiber. Overcooking breaks down the sulfur compounds in cabbage and can create a permeating odor. To remedy this, cook cabbage just until it is tender, using stainless steel pots and pans.

- Almost all **cauliflower** grown in the United States comes from the Salinas Valley in California. Its florets are actually undeveloped white flower buds. Cauliflower is high in vitamin C, folate, and fiber. Choose cauliflower that is creamy white with firm, compact florets and bright green leaves. Nix cauliflower that has lots of dark spots and wilted, yellowish leaves. Mashed cauliflower is a vitamin-packed alternative to mashed potatoes.

- **Collard greens** are high in beta-carotene, calcium, and fiber. They are fibrous and tough and can require cooking times of up to one hour. They should be washed several times to remove all dirt and grit. To save the nutrients that are leached out, add the liquid left over after cooking to soups and stews.

- **Kale** is a source of vitamins A, C, and K and calcium, potassium, and fiber. The term "kale" is derived from *coles* or *caulis*, used by Greeks and Romans to refer to a cabbage-like group of plants. It is a primitive cabbage that has been around for thousands of years. Raw or lightly steamed kale adds texture, color, and flavor to many dishes and can be used as a substitute for other greens. And at about thirty-five calories per cup with fiber to fill you up, it's not a bad food to aid in weight loss!

- **Mustard greens** are a source of beta-carotene, fiber, calcium, iron, and potassium. They can be eaten either raw or cooked and are available in the winter when most vegetables are not in season. Store unwashed mustard greens in plastic bags in the refrigerator, and they will keep for about three days. As with arugula and watercress, spice up salads with a peppery flavor by adding mustard greens.

- **Swiss chard** is high in vitamins A, K, and C and potassium and fiber (the leaves being more nutritious than the root). The leaves are always green, but the stalks are either red or yellow. It is a sturdy green, but it has a more delicate flavor than other greens such as kale or turnip greens. If using in salads, choose fresh, young chard.

- **Turnip greens** are a great source of vitamins A, K, and C and calcium and fiber for only about twenty calories per cup. Turnip greens are high in oxalates that can accumulate in the body. You may want to avoid eating them if you have a history of kidney stones or gall bladder problems. (Eating them with a calcium-rich food or beverage can help avoid problems.) To spice up your turnip greens, eliminate extra fat by substituting onions, pepper, and other fat-free, low-calorie extras for the higher-fat items such as salt pork.

- **Watercress** is high in vitamins A, C, and K and very low in calories (about four calories per cup). A peer-reviewed study reported in the *American Journal of Clinical Nutrition* found that daily consumption of watercress may reduce DNA damage to blood cells and may lower the risk of cancer to many parts of the body. As with mustard greens and arugula, watercress can add a peppery flavoring to salads and other foods.

Dairy

(serving size = one cup milk or yogurt, 1½ ounces cheese,
two ounces processed cheese)

- A study tracked the diets of 75,000 middle-aged and older adults for ten years. Daily average consumption of four servings of low-fat cheeses, yogurts, and milk lowered their risk of stroke by 12 percent. Full-fat dairy products were not associated with lower risk, possibly because of the counteracting effect of higher LDL (bad) cholesterol that may result.

- Include low-fat or fat-free milk and/or yogurt in smoothies. Even if you don't care for the taste of dairy, a smoothie with added fruit, cereal, or a dash of vanilla extract will make for a delicious-tasting concoction with which you can truly "toast to your health."

- If you are lactose intolerant, try taking a commercial lactose enzyme with your dairy, or eat yogurt that refers to "live and active bacteria" on its label—this means most of the milk sugar has been predigested (see more on yogurt as a food in this chapter). Also, you can consume fermented dairy products such as hard cheeses, cottage cheese, or kefir (see more on kefir as a food in this chapter).

Fish, Cold-Water

(serving size = 3-4 ounces)

- Cold-water fish contain omega-3 fats rich in eicosapentaenoic acid (EPA) and docosahexaenoic acid (DHA). EPA and DHA are believed to provide the health benefits attributed to omega-3 fats from fish. The type of omega-3 fat found in plant foods, such as flax seed and various nuts, although having certain health benefits and providing the essential alpha-linolenic (ALA) fatty acid, do not contain EPA and DHA. Your body does, however, partially convert ALA to EPA and DHA. The American Heart Association recommends healthy people eat fish twice a week.

- Getting omega-3 fat from fish is the recommended way, but if you do not eat fish or other foods rich in omega-3s, you should consider taking an omega-3 supplement of 500 milligrams per day. If you have had a heart attack, you may benefit from doubling the dose to 500 mg twice daily. Check with your doctor before taking a supplement, to see if it is advisable for you, given your health condition and any medications you may be taking.

- Predator fish (e.g., shark, swordfish, tilefish, king mackerel, and albacore tuna) should be consumed in limited quantities, especially you are if pregnant or breastfeeding, as they contain the largest quantities of mercury. Fish with safer amounts include shellfish, canned fish (especially light tuna), and smaller fish. Pregnant or breastfeeding women and young children should eat no more than six ounces of albacore or twelve ounces of light tuna per week.

- It is recommended that you eat at least eight ounces of fish twice a week to get optimal health benefits. Pregnant or breastfeeding women can safely eat up to twelve ounces per week of fish that are not high in mercury.

- **Anchovies**, averaging one to four inches in length, are in the herring family and swim in warm water. They have an intense fishy and salty taste, so that people either love them or loathe them. They were very special to the Roman Empire, however, as they were used to make a condiment (garum) that rivaled the finest perfumes in price. To eliminate saltiness, soak anchovies in water for about half an hour, then pat them dry with paper towels. Spice up your recipes with them; they are particularly good in a Caesar salad.

- **Halibut** is a flat fish that can grow to eight feet long and weigh more than 500 pounds, although most of the larger variety are harvested at fifty to 100 pounds. It has a sweet flavor and firm, flaky meat. A smaller variety, called chicken Halibut and weighing in at about ten pounds, is the tastiest. Since halibut is low in oil content, it's a good fish to marinate or brush with olive oil prior to cooking.

- **Herring** has been a regular food source since before 3000 BC. The two main types are Atlantic herring, growing up to eighteen inches, and Pacific herring, growing up to fifteen inches. The shiny, silver-colored fish are eaten in many ways, including raw, fermented, pickled, and salted. Because of its high oil content, herring is a good fish to be smoked.

- The prominent stripes on the backs of **mackerels** help them align with adjacent fish, match their speed, and signal changes of position. This helps them swim together when schooling from one location to another. As with most fish, when purchasing, select one with clear, glassy eyes, red gills, and a firm texture. The firmness of mackerel allows for easy grilling. Grill on each side for about five minutes. Wrap in foil for a lighter taste.

- The size of a **salmon** usually indicates its age. Chinook salmon are the longest living, at up to nine years, and weigh over 100 pounds. Although probably outweighed by its health benefits, farmed salmon has been found to have high levels of toxic man-made chemicals. Therefore, it may be more reassuring to purchase wild salmon rather than farm raised, particularly for pregnant or breastfeeding women.

- **Sardines** are small, silvery fish that travel in large schools and are related to herring. The term *sardine* is believed to have originated in the fifteenth century. Sardines were abundant around the island Sardinia in the Mediterranean. Eating a can of sardines, loaded with omega-3 fats, will also give you more calcium than a glass of milk. Be sure to eat the whole sardine, as the calcium source is its spine.

- Although the largest recorded **swordfish** weighed in at 1,200 pounds, the average swordfish caught commercially weighs between 200 and 330 pounds. The snout protrudes into a sword that measures at least one-third of the body length and is flat, pointed, and very sharp. Cook swordfish until opaque with a bit of pink or ivory in the center. Remove the skin before eating, as it is tough and not very tasty. Try adding a little lemon juice during cooking to spice up the taste a bit.

- **Lake trout**, members of the salmon family, are the largest trout in North America, with sizes that vary according to the body of water in which they are found. The largest catch on record is 102 pounds, caught in Lake Athabasca, Saskatchewan, in 1961. The average lake trout caught commercially weighs between four and five pounds. Trout that is two to four pounds is best to prepare, as larger ones do not taste as good.

- **Albacore tuna** is the only type that can be marketed as "white meat tuna" in the United States. It is a relatively small tuna and is the major source of canned tuna. To get some fruit and veggies in addition to the protein and omega-3 fat provided by tuna, create a tuna salad for lunch or snack. Empty a can of tuna into a bowl and add sliced grapes, celery, apples, diced bell peppers, low-fat mayonnaise, and anything else your heart desires. Then put it on crackers, in a sandwich, or just eat it straight up!

Flax Seed

(serving size = one tablespoon)

- Flax seeds contain omega-3 fats known as alpha-linolenic acid. This type of omega-3 fat is different from the omega-3 fats found in cold-water fish. Flax and other plant omega-3 fats, although having health benefits, convey smaller health benefits than those from fish.

- Both fish and plant omega-3s are essential fats, meaning you must get them from food because your body doesn't make them.

- Sprinkle flax seed meal on salads or hot and cold cereals or add to casseroles. It should be stored in opaque packaging, kept refrigerated, away from light, and be used within forty-five days.

Garlic

(serving size = to taste)

- Garlic's active compounds can lose their potency with time and processing, so it is difficult to estimate the amount of garlic one should consume to reap its benefits. However, the World Health Organization's guidelines for general health is a daily dose of two to five grams of fresh garlic (about one clove), 0.4 to 1.2 grams of dried powder, 2 to 5 milligrams of garlic oil, or 300 to 1,000 milligrams of garlic extract.

- There haven't been many vampires spotted recently, but that doesn't mean garlic still can't have some practical use as a repellent. If you garden, spray a garlic mixture on plants to keep the locals (deer, rabbits, and other four-legged vegetarians) from chomping your vittles before you get a chance to.

Ginseng

(serving size = to taste)

- There are many types of ginseng, but Panax ginseng of the Asiatic variety is most commonly used in America. Although we grow ginseng in America (about 90 percent of it in Wisconsin), we export most of it and import Korean ginseng for our use. Panax is derived from the Greek word *panakeia*, meaning "universal remedy." Besides its purported medicinal uses, it is also used throughout the world to make soaps, cosmetics, toothpaste, chewing gum, soft drinks, tea, candy, cigarettes, and to flavor beverages. Many believe that the older the ginseng root, the longer it will enhance life. One 400-year-old Chinese ginseng root is documented to have been sold for $10,000 an ounce!

- Most studies are inconclusive as to the benefits of ginseng. The effective dosage for type 2 diabetes is 200 mg per day, and for erectile dysfunction 900 mg three times a day.

- If you take Panax ginseng for memory, use it in combination with ginkgo leaf extract. While it is not found to improve memory alone, there is evidence of effectiveness from using the two in tandem.

- If you do take it, the Commission E (Germany's regulator agency for herbs) recommends no more than one to two grams (1,000 to 2,000 milligrams) daily of the root for no more than three months (long-term use could be harmful, due to its hormone-like effects). Ginseng in babies has been linked to poisoning that can be fatal. The safety in older children is not known, so is to be considered as probably unsafe. Pregnant women should not take ginseng because animal studies show it leads to birth defects. Little is known about its effects on breastfeeding, so it should be avoided in this instance as well. Most people should check with a health professional before taking ginseng, as there are many contraindications with other medicines and disease states.

Grains, Whole

(serving size = one ounce—one cup cold cereal; ½ cup cooked rice, pasta, cooked cereal; one slice bread)

- A whole grain consists of bran, germ, and endosperm and is rich in fiber and several vitamins and minerals. Refined/processed grains don't have the bran and germ and lack fiber and many other nutrients of the whole grain (about 80 percent of phytonutrients are lost during processing). When shopping for whole grain foods, such as breads and cereals, don't be misled by front-of-package labeling. Terms such as multigrain don't necessarily mean whole grain but merely that the product consists of more than one type of grain. It could be that several refined grains were used. Read the ingredients (usually in small print somewhere on package) and see if whole grain is the first or second item listed. Then look at the nutrition facts label and see how much fiber there is in a serving.

- To avoid refined flour and get some fiber into your life, try making homemade pizza with whole grain crust or flapjacks with whole grain pancake mix. Your digestive system will love you for it!

Grapes

(serving size = ½ cup—about fifteen grapes)

- Resveratrol is the most well-known phytonutrient in grapes and red wine. It is found in the skins of grapes, with dark grapes (especially the Concord variety) having the highest amounts. You can be a teetotaler and still get your supply of resveratrol. In addition to red wine, you can get it from grape juice and the grapes themselves.

- Instead of syrup, spread grape jam on waffles or pancakes to provide a bit of sweetness. Drink a mixture of Concord grape juice and kefir to get the health benefits of resveratrol from the grapes and probiotics from the kefir. It's a good way to get your system revved up to start the day!

Green Leafy Vegetables

(serving size = one cup raw leaves, ½ cup cooked)

- At the top of the list for nutritional value among the leafy greens is kale. If you are concerned about your vision and the prospect of contracting macular degeneration as you get older, this is the veggie for you. Kale tops the list with the vision-saving phytonutrient lutein, having 11,900 micrograms. But for all you Popeye fans, spinach comes in a close second with 10,200 micrograms.

- Keep packages of prewashed leafy greens on hand as the foundation for a salad. Having other veggies, such as broccoli florets, baby carrots, nuts, previously sliced cucumber and bell pepper, etc. makes salad prep quick and easy when arriving home from work or school.

Kefir

(serving size = eight ounces)

- Kefir is a fermented yogurt-like drink originating in Russia. It is rich with probiotic (friendly) bacteria, providing numerous health benefits.

- If you don't like plain kefir's sour taste, you can either purchase the flavored kind or mix the unflavored with fruit juice.

Lentils

(serving size = ½ cup)

- Lentils, members of the legume family, are lens-shaped seeds that are estimated to have been in the human diet for more than 9,000 years. They are high in protein, folate, iron, potassium, and fiber and low in fat. Although high in protein, they lack the essential amino acids methionine and cysteine and should be mixed with grains to be a complete protein source.

- Lentils do not need to be presoaked like other legumes. Brown lentils, the least expensive, get mushy when cooked and should be used in soups, but green lentils stay firm and can be used for salads. Red and orange lentils cook in about twenty minutes, whereas brown and green ones take about forty-five minutes.

Mushrooms

(serving size = ½ cup)

- Although bananas are often touted as the premier source of potassium (why they're used by so many athletes), one portabella mushroom has more potassium than a banana.

- One reason why mushrooms can grow in the dark is that they have no chlorophyll and don't need sunshine to grow.

- A thick grilled portabella mushroom can be a pretty good substitute for meat, particularly in a sandwich. Mushrooms can be added to most anything—casseroles, omelets, sandwiches, pizza, or salads, to name just a few.

Nuts

(serving size = one ounce)

- Nuts are high in fat and calories and should replace the saturated fat in your diet, rather than as an addition. A small handful (about one ounce) a day is enough to lower your risk of heart disease.

- Add nuts to oatmeal, pancakes, salads, yogurt, or an ice cream sundae for extra crunch, protein, and taste.

Oil, Canola

(serving size = one tablespoon)

- Limited scientific evidence suggests that eating about 1½ tablespoons (nineteen grams) of canola oil daily may reduce the risk of heart disease.

- Canola oil has a light texture and neutral taste, giving it versatility. It can be used to bake, stir-fry, or fry at medium-high temperatures.

Oil, Corn

(serving size = one tablespoon)

- Very limited and preliminary scientific evidence suggest that eating about one tablespoon (sixteen grams) of corn oil daily may reduce the risk of heart disease.

- Popularly used in margarines, corn oil can also be used for baking and frying at medium temperatures.

Oil, Olive

(serving size = one tablespoon)

- Limited scientific evidence suggests that eating about two table-spoons (twenty-three grams) of olive oil daily may reduce the risk of heart disease.

- There are many varieties of olive oil—extra virgin, virgin, extra light, and refined. Extra virgin is the most common; it comes from the first press of the olives and contains the most polyphe-nols (phytonutrients found to be good for health). Drizzle some on bread instead of margarine, or mix a little with vinegar for a heart-healthy salad dressing.

Onions

(serving size = ½ cup)

- Onions are an organosulfur vegetable, and the sulfuric compounds are what make us cry like babies when preparing them. To avoid crying jags, chill the onion or run cold water over it before cut-ting. Cut into the root end of the onion last.

- Onions can be added to many types of foods for flavor enhance-ment, allowing for less fat and salt to be used.

Peanuts

(serving size = one ounce)

- Peanuts are not tree nuts but legumes. Although they are a differ-ent classification from other nuts, they have almost all the qualities and characteristics of true tree nuts.

- If you don't like eating just plain nuts, eat the butters. Peanut but-ter is made of over 90 percent ground peanuts and provides the health benefits of raw peanuts. And to get even more of the health benefits, boil peanuts to enhance their antioxidant availability.

Pepper, Black

(serving size = to taste)

- Black pepper is a pungent spice that was first grown in southern India more than 2,000 years ago. The pepper plant, a smooth, woody vine grown in hot, humid tropical climates, can reach thirty-three feet in length.

- Studies showing pepper's ability to block fat cell creation were done in the lab in petri dishes, not on humans, so take this quality with a grain of salt (pun intended!). If nothing else, pepper is a good substitute for salt to spice up food, especially for those who are cutting back on salt consumption.

- Since its flavor diminishes during cooking, pepper should be added either near the end of cooking or at the table.

Peppers, Bell

(serving size = ½ cup)

- Bell peppers come in a variety of colors, depending on their stage of ripeness. Green bell peppers are the least ripe, followed by yellow, orange, and red. While all are plentiful with nutrients, the reds are the powerhouse, having the most time to ripen on the vine.

- Cut up bell peppers and add them to salads or omelets. But don't cut them too much ahead of time, or they'll lose their vitamin C punch.

Peppers, Hot

(serving size = to taste)

- Peppers, although considered by most to be a vegetable, are technically fruits.

- Eating moderate amounts of capsaicin, the ingredient making peppers hot, is enough to reap the health benefits. One weight loss study on humans used only one gram, or half a teaspoon, and it worked best for those who hadn't eaten it regularly prior to the study. While some evidence exists that hot peppers may lower risk of stomach cancer, research also indicates that eating excessive amounts may be linked to stomach cancer. And although it does not cause stomach ulcers, capsaicin can make them worse. Therefore, as with most other things, moderation is the key. The capsaicin oil is located in the pepper's ribs and seeds.

- If the burn is too much, grab a glass of milk or other dairy product with some fat, not water. Capsaicin, the substance in peppers that causes thermal discomfort, dissolves in fat, and milk contains a fat-dissolving substance that neutralizes the capsaicin.

- Fresh chili peppers should feel firm and have a smooth skin. Generally, the more pointed the tips, the hotter the chili pepper. There are numerous types of chilis, each conveying various degrees of heat.

- The **habanero** brings more heat than any other chili pepper. It is one of the hottest peppers in the world and registers as about 100 times hotter than the jalapeño! Always use gloves when preparing habaneros, as they can literally burn your skin. Needless to say, keep them away from your eyes and nose. (If your eyes begin watering, be careful not to rub them with the hands you used to touch the peppers!)

- **Jalapeño** peppers are the most common chili pepper in America. They can provide a spicy-hot punch to foods. How much punch can vary, however, according to the cultivation and preparation methods used.

Plantains

(serving size = one medium, ½ cup)

- Plantains are different from bananas in that they are firmer and less sweet and need to be cooked. They don't need to be ripe but can be cooked at all stages of ripeness—green, yellow, or black. They are sources of vitamin C, fiber, and potassium.

- To peel a plantain, cut off its ends, slit the skin from one end to the other, then peel off the skin sideways. If you are not cooking it immediately, place it in salt water to keep it from becoming discolored.

Popcorn

(serving size = about two cups popped)

- Popcorn is the only snack that is 100 percent unprocessed whole grain—you can't get more than that! Just one serving provides 70 percent of the daily recommended amount of whole grains.

- Much of the popcorn that you purchase outside of the home— think movie popcorn—can have 1,200 calories or more (before adding all that fake butter)! So either get some low-fat microwave popcorn or pop your own. Invest in an air popper. If you want to jazz it up a bit, you can add some spices to your taste—Mrs. Dash, cinnamon, pepper, etc. To make it stick better, give it a *small* shot of spray cooking oil (butter flavored, if you like).

Prunes

(serving size = ¼ cup)

- The prune industry has attempted to give prunes a facelift by marketing them as dried plums. No matter what you call them, prunes or dried plums, they pack a nutritional punch and are definitely one of the good guys to include in your diet.

- Prunes by themselves are a healthy, convenient on-the-go snack. Pit-free prunes can also be blended into smoothies to add a touch of fiber and sweetness.

Raisins

(serving size = ¼ cup)

- Raisins (dried grapes) have antioxidant and anti-inflammatory properties that can bestow generous health benefits. They also contribute fiber, iron, and various other nutrients to the diet.

- Add plenty of raisins to oatmeal raisin cookies for loads of nutrients, including soluble fiber for heart health. Sweeten your hot oatmeal cereal by mixing in a quarter cup of raisins instead of sugar.

Rosemary

(serving size = to taste)

- A member of the mint family and full of antioxidants, one of the theories of rosemary's etymology derives from the legend that the Virgin Mary spread her blue cloak over a white-blossomed rosemary bush and the flowers turned blue. The bush then became known as the "Rose of Mary."

- The Greeks believed rosemary boosted brainpower and memory, so they wove it into their hair. This may not be so far fetched, as a study reported in the journal *Therapeutic Advances in Psychopharmacology* indicated that smelling the fragrance increased speed and accuracy on mathematics tests.

- Use ground rosemary leaves for meats, grains, potatoes, marinades, and soups; put the woody stems in the grill to provide aroma to your foods.

Soy
(serving size = ½ cup beans, tofu; eight ounces milk)

- Studies have indicated that soy foods and beverages may provide health benefits, from lessening hot flashes in menopausal women to lowering the risk of heart disease. Supplements, not soy foods, were used in the studies. You should be able to derive these benefits from two servings of soy food per day—about two eight-ounce glasses of soy milk, seven ounces of tofu, or half a cup of edamame.

- There are a variety of soy product lines for just about anything you might want—yogurt substitute, meatless sandwich patties, cheese substitute, soymilk, etc. If you want to cut out saturated fat, think soy burger or soy cheese. You'll be getting plenty of protein with these soy choices.

Sweet Potatoes
(serving size = ½ cup)

- Sweet potatoes are an excellent source of vitamin A and a good source of vitamins B6, C, and E along with folate and potassium. They are high in fiber too.

- Sweet potatoes are very tasty and don't need to be doctored up as much as regular potatoes do. If you do, though, be careful to avoid making it into a fat bomb. Use a light margarine of the variety that has other health benefits—added omega-3 fats or plant sterols can lower triglycerides or cholesterol.

Tea

(serving size = six to eight fluid ounces)

- Only teas derived from the Camellia sinensis shrub are considered true teas—black, green, white, oolong and Pu-erh. Herbal teas are from various roots, leaves, etc., and have fewer antioxidant compounds than true teas.

- Adding citrus juice (orange, lemon, grapefruit, or lime) to tea has been found to increase its main health-providing substances (catechins).

Tomatoes

(serving size = one medium, ½ cup)

- Should be cooked to release the antioxidant lycopene from the cell wall.

- Cook with a healthy oil, such as olive oil, as lycopene (a carotenoid) is more readily absorbed when eaten with fat.

- When preparing a tomato-based dish, such as spaghetti sauce, heat in an iron skillet. The iron skillet tends to leach iron into whatever food is being cooked in it. This is especially true for acidic substances, such as tomato sauces.

Turmeric

(serving size = to taste)

- A culinary spice, turmeric is the main ingredient in Indian curries. It is used to add color to butter, margarine, cheese, and mustard, and to add tint to cotton, silk, paper, and cosmetics. It has been used as a food preservative and to make pickles.

- Turmeric, and its chief component, curcumin, have been used for 4,000 years to treat conditions from infections and inflammation to digestive problems and some types of cancer. Use in traditional Chinese and Indian medicine is documented from the seventh century. Various studies, conducted in either test tubes, animals, or humans, have provided evidence of its benefits for indigestion, ulcerative colitis, stomach ulcers, osteoarthritis, heart disease, liver damage, and some cancers. There is no standardized dose for turmeric, but recommendations for dried turmeric may vary from one teaspoon daily to one at each meal.

- If you are taking blood-thinning medication, drugs to reduce stomach acid, or diabetes medications, check with your doctor before using turmeric or curcumin supplements, as they can increase the effects of blood thinners, may interfere with the action of medicines taken to decrease stomach acidity, and can strengthen the effects of diabetes medications, increasing the risk of hypoglycemia. Pregnant or breastfeeding women should also check with their physicians before using this herbal supplement.

- Turmeric powder is bitter and may be distasteful to some people. However, diluting it by adding a couple of teaspoons to a large container of soup, stew, or casserole can make the taste subtle enough to appease the palate. Add pepper to your dish to enhance the absorption of turmeric and curcumin, both of which are otherwise poorly absorbed. Piperine is the substance in black pepper that increases absorption. This is why both turmeric and pepper are used together in many Indian foods. Look for piperine or black pepper extract as an ingredient when shopping for a curcumin or turmeric supplement.

Ugli Fruit

(serving size = ½ cup)

- The name says it all! Look for what looks like a grapefruit with a wrinkled, greenish-yellow skin. It has a sweet taste, although slightly less so than an orange.

- Although all seasonal varieties are sweet and juicy, the fruit available in December and January is tastier than what appears later in the season.

Watermelon

(serving size = ½ cup)

- Watermelon is the fruit that is really a vegetable. It is part of the cucumber and squash family. It contains 92 percent water and 8 percent sugar—thus its name.

- The *Guinness Book of World Records*' largest watermelon was 262 pounds.

- When choosing a watermelon, thump the melon with your middle finger. It should produce a deep, rich thudding sound. Although they will ripen a little at room temperature, melons picked before they are ripe will never attain full flavor.

Wheat Germ

(serving size = two tablespoons)

- The "germ" in wheat germ is short for germination. Wheat germ is the embryo of the wheat kernel that grows into a new plant.

- It is the most nutrient-rich part of the kernel. Per serving it provides about forty-five calories, three grams of protein, two grams of fiber, polyunsaturated fats, essential omega-3 fats and is loaded with other nutrients, such as iron, zinc, potassium, and many B vitamins.

- Added to smoothies, hot or cold cereals, salads, or soups, wheat germ will add some "nutrient punch" to your diet.

- Wheat germ should be kept refrigerated, as the polyunsaturated fats can become rancid with storage.

Wine, Red
(serving size = five ounces)

- If you don't already drink alcohol, you needn't start. The health components of red wine can be acquired from dark grapes and their juices and jams. If you do indulge, do so in moderation to avoid health problems associated with alcohol. No more than one drink per day for women and two for men is considered moderate. (Sorry ladies, but men have more alcohol dehydrogenase to metabolize alcohol more efficiently and clear it from their bodies faster.) One drink of wine equals five ounces.

- If you do imbibe occasionally, you might not have to shell out so much of your mad money to get a wine to enjoy. A Penn State study revealed, not surprisingly, that professional wine tasters appear to have a much more sensitive sense of taste than most. So if you want to be a wine snob, that's fine, but you might be able to indulge your palate a lot more economically than you think!

- Concord grapes contain the most resveratrol, the substance in grapes and red wine most frequently studied for its health benefits.

Yogurt

(serving size = one cup)

- When purchasing yogurt, look on the container for the term "contains live and active cultures" or something to this effect. This means the health-providing probiotic bacteria are viable and can be of benefit to you.

- There are numerous types of yogurt from which to choose, including yogurt with fiber and high-protein Greek yogurt. It's a great snack, and of course it is an excellent addition to a smoothie. And if you're lactose intolerant, you should be able to digest yogurt that contains live and active cultures, as they will have predigested the milk sugars.

General Information

- Many of the foods listed contain antioxidants. Antioxidants neutralize free radicals, substances that can damage cells and lead to cancer and other chronic diseases. These phytonutrients found in plant foods are the closest we've come to discovering a fountain of youth.

- Rinse and then eat the skins of fruits and vegetables, as many of their nutrients are found there.

- Carotenoids are fat-soluble and are best absorbed with fat in a meal. Chopping, pureeing, and cooking carotenoid-containing vegetables in oil can increase absorption of their special disease-fighting nutrients.

- Evidence from numerous scientific studies suggests that the thousands of nontraditional nutrients we are finding in plant foods do not act in isolation but are complementary. Supplements have not provided the same health benefits as eating a variety of plant-derived foods.

Note:

Information used to create this listing was obtained from meta-analyses of scientifically sound, peer-reviewed studies whenever possible. (A meta-analysis is a compilation of many studies.) Much of the scientific evidence supporting the health benefits reported is limited and preliminary. Although evidence was derived from human studies whenever possible, a considerable proportion was obtained from studies conducted either with animals or in vitro (outside of a living entity). The science of human nutrition is in its early stages, and although there are many promising health benefits of foods and food components, time, funding, ethical concerns and other factors have as yet prevented more extensive human studies. Another reason for not having more definitive scientific evidence lies with the difficulty of isolating a particular food or food substance in the human diet and determining that it is responsible for a specific health benefit, given all the other competing diet and lifestyle factors. Scientists also believe that many foods and nutrients work synergistically, which is why many studies reveal the benefits of foods and diets but not the individual nutrients in supplement form. Therefore, the safest nutritional recommendation at this point would be to eat a variety of fruits, vegetables, whole grains, low-fat dairy and dairy alternatives, and other foods and beverages that are recommended by expert health agencies, such as the USDA at http://www.choosemyplate.gov/.

ABOUT THE AUTHOR

DAVID RATH, MA, RDN, LD is a registered dietitian nutritionist and owner of David Rath Nutrition, Inc., in Little Rock, Arkansas. David counsels patients for nutrition-related health problems, weight loss, general wellness, and sports nutrition. He also provides wellness services to organizations that want to ensure a healthy workforce, frequently speaks to various community groups, and appears as a nutrition expert in print and broadcast media.

A member of the Academy of Nutrition and Dietetics, David also belongs to the Weight Management Dietetic Practice Group and the Sports, Cardiovascular and Wellness Dietetic Practice Group. He has a Certificate of Training in Adult Weight Management from the Academy of Nutrition and Dietetics and the Commission on Dietetic Registration.

Previously, David was Nutrition Chief for the Arkansas Department of Health. He also served on the Arkansas Governor's Council on Fitness and was chair of the nutrition committee of the Arkansas Coalition for Obesity Prevention and served on its executive committee. David was on the executive board of the Arkansas Food Policy Council and chaired its nutrition committee. He has presented at numerous national and state conferences and has been published in the Centers for Disease Control and Prevention's *Journal of Chronic Diseases*. David, due to his community service, also had the honor of being chosen as a torchbearer for the Salt Lake City 2000 Olympics.

Made in the USA
Columbia, SC
01 April 2018